Christoph Eisenegger

The modulation of human brain function to study decision making

Christoph Eisenegger

The modulation of human brain function to study decision making

Psychopharmacology and transcranial magnetic stimulation as tools to investigate individual and social decision making behaviour in humans

Südwestdeutscher Verlag für Hochschulschriften

Impressum/Imprint (nur für Deutschland/ only for Germany)
Bibliografische Information der Deutschen Nationalbibliothek: Die Deutsche Nationalbibliothek verzeichnet diese Publikation in der Deutschen Nationalbibliografie; detaillierte bibliografische Daten sind im Internet über http://dnb.d-nb.de abrufbar.

Alle in diesem Buch genannten Marken und Produktnamen unterliegen warenzeichen-, marken- oder patentrechtlichem Schutz bzw. sind Warenzeichen oder eingetragene Warenzeichen der jeweiligen Inhaber. Die Wiedergabe von Marken, Produktnamen, Gebrauchsnamen, Handelsnamen, Warenbezeichnungen u.s.w. in diesem Werk berechtigt auch ohne besondere Kennzeichnung nicht zu der Annahme, dass solche Namen im Sinne der Warenzeichen- und Markenschutzgesetzgebung als frei zu betrachten wären und daher von jedermann benutzt werden dürften.

Verlag: Südwestdeutscher Verlag für Hochschulschriften Aktiengesellschaft & Co. KG
Dudweiler Landstr. 99, 66123 Saarbrücken, Deutschland
Telefon +49 681 37 20 271-1, Telefax +49 681 37 20 271-0
Email: info@svh-verlag.de
Zugl.: Zürich, Eidgenössische Technische Hochschule Zürich, Diss., 2009

Herstellung in Deutschland:
Schaltungsdienst Lange o.H.G., Berlin
Books on Demand GmbH, Norderstedt
Reha GmbH, Saarbrücken
Amazon Distribution GmbH, Leipzig
ISBN: 978-3-8381-1718-8

Imprint (only for USA, GB)
Bibliographic information published by the Deutsche Nationalbibliothek: The Deutsche Nationalbibliothek lists this publication in the Deutsche Nationalbibliografie; detailed bibliographic data are available in the Internet at http://dnb.d-nb.de.

Any brand names and product names mentioned in this book are subject to trademark, brand or patent protection and are trademarks or registered trademarks of their respective holders. The use of brand names, product names, common names, trade names, product descriptions etc. even without a particular marking in this works is in no way to be construed to mean that such names may be regarded as unrestricted in respect of trademark and brand protection legislation and could thus be used by anyone.

Publisher: Südwestdeutscher Verlag für Hochschulschriften Aktiengesellschaft & Co. KG
Dudweiler Landstr. 99, 66123 Saarbrücken, Germany
Phone +49 681 37 20 271-1, Fax +49 681 37 20 271-0
Email: info@svh-verlag.de

Printed in the U.S.A.
Printed in the U.K. by (see last page)
ISBN: 978-3-8381-1718-8

Copyright © 2010 by the author and Südwestdeutscher Verlag für Hochschulschriften Aktiengesellschaft & Co. KG and licensors
All rights reserved. Saarbrücken 2010

Contents

I Theoretical Part — 1

1 Introduction to the topic — 3

2 Neuromodulatory approaches to study decision making — 5
- 2.1 Brain stimulation — 5
  - 2.1.1 Transcranial magnetic stimulation — 6
  - 2.1.2 Summary — 8
- 2.2 Neuropharmacological modulation — 10
  - 2.2.1 Dopaminergic system — 11
  - 2.2.2 Pharmacogenetics and behaviour — 15
  - 2.2.3 Pathological gambling in Parkinson's disease patients — 16
  - 2.2.4 Summary — 18
- 2.3 Neuroendocrine modulation — 18
  - 2.3.1 The androgen system — 19
  - 2.3.2 Neuroendocrinology — 23
  - 2.3.3 Behavioural effects of testosterone — 26
  - 2.3.4 Social behaviour in humans — 27
  - 2.3.5 Summary — 32

II Empirical Part — 33

3 Study 1: Time-course of "off-line" prefrontal rTMS effects – a PET study — 35
- 3.1 Contributions — 35
- 3.2 Introduction — 35
- 3.3 Materials and methods — 37
  - 3.3.1 Subjects — 37
  - 3.3.2 PET procedures — 37

		3.3.3	Location of the target region	38
		3.3.4	rTMS procedure	38
		3.3.5	Image analysis	38
		3.3.6	Region of interest analysis	39
		3.3.7	Masked correlation analysis	40
	3.4	Results	41
		3.4.1	Time-course of "off-line" prefrontal rTMS effects on rCBF	41
	3.5	Discussion	43
	3.6	Supplementary material	47
	3.7	Comments on Study 1	50
		3.7.1	"Off-line" rTMS of the DLPFC and social decision making . . .	50
		3.7.2	Virtual lesion	51

4 Study 2: DRD4 polymorphism predicts the effect of L-DOPA on gambling behaviour   53

	4.1	Contributions	53
	4.2	Introduction	53
	4.3	Results	54
	4.4	Discussion	56
	4.5	Methods	57
		4.5.1	Subjects	57
		4.5.2	Experimental procedure	57
		4.5.3	Genotyping	58
		4.5.4	Subject grouping according to the DRD4 exon III VNTR polymorphism genotype	59
		4.5.5	Gambling task	60
		4.5.6	Measures of drug related side effects	60
		4.5.7	Statistical analysis	62
	4.6	Comments on Study 2	63
		4.6.1	Motor repetitive behaviour	63
		4.6.2	DRD4 modulation	64
			Prefrontal cortex and impulse control	64
			Striatum and reward sensitivity	66
		4.6.3	Self-reported impulsivity and gambling behaviour	67
		4.6.4	Specificity of L-DOPA effects	68
		4.6.5	Combining fMRI with neuropharmacological modulation	69
		4.6.6	Does one gene determine one behaviour?	70
		4.6.7	Implications for clinical practice in psychiatry	71

   Treatment of Parkinson's disease 72
   The dopamine hypothesis of ADHD: revision necessary? 75

5 Study 3: Prejudice and truth: the effect of testosterone administration on bargaining behaviour   **77**
 5.1 Contributions 77
 5.2 Introduction and results 77
 5.3 Discussion 84
 5.4 Methods 87
   5.4.1 Subjects 87
   5.4.2 Experimental procedure 87
   5.4.3 Salivary measurements 88
   5.4.4 Questionnaires 89
   5.4.5 Statistical analysis 90
   5.4.6 *Post-hoc* online survey 90
 5.5 Comments on Study 3 93
   5.5.1 External validity of economic games 93
   5.5.2 Testosterone rules...? 95
   5.5.3 Specificity of testosterone effects 97
      Is testosterone a *pro*hormone? 97
   5.5.4 Suppression of the reproductive axis 98

III   General conclusions   **101**

IV   Appendix   **107**

List of abbreviations

^{11}C L-DOPA	^{11}C labelled L-DOPA PET tracer	65
^{18}F L-DOPA	^{18}F labelled L-DOPA PET tracer	65
17-β-HSD	17-β-hydroxysteroid dehydrogenase	20
5-HT	5-hydroxy tryptamine or serotonin	11
5-HTP	5-hydroxy tryptophan	11
5-HTTPP	Serotonin transporter polymorphism	15
7R allele	7 repeats allele	13
AADC	Aromatic amino-acid decarboxylase	11
ACC	Anterior cingulate cortex	10
ACTH	Adrenocorticotropic hormone	20
ADH	Aldehyd-dehydrogenase	11
ADHD	Attention deficit hyperactivity disorder	14
ANOVA	Analysis of variance	40
AR	Androgen receptor	21
BA	Brodmann area	7
BBB	Blood brain barrier	11
BDNF	Brain derived neurotrophic factor	70
BOLD signal	Blood-oxygen level dependent signal	69
c_{max}	Maximum serum or salivary concentration	98
cAMP	Cyclic adenosine-monophosphate	12
CNS	Central nervous system	22
COMT	Catechol-O-methyl transferase	11
CORT	Cortisol	23
CRH	Corticotropin releasing hormone	23
CSF	Cerebrospinal fluid	11
DA	Dopamine	4
DAT	Dopamine transporter	75

DAT polym.	DAT 40 base-pair VNTR polymorphism	67
DBH	Dopamine-β-hydroxylase	11
DHEA	Dihydroepiandrosterone	20
DHT	Dihydrotestosterone	20
DLPFC	Dorsolateral prefrontal cortex	6
DNA	Desoxynucleic acid	21
DOPAC	Dihydroxyphenylacetic acid	11
DRD2 polym.	Taq1A DA receptor D2 polymorphism	15
DRD4 polym.	DA receptor D4 VNTR polymorphism	13
E2	17-β-estradiol	20
EEG	Electroencephalography	7
ER-α	Estrogen receptor alpha	21
ER-β	Estrogen receptor beta	21
fMRI	Functional magnetic resonance imaging	7
FSH	Follicle stimulating hormone	24
FWHM	Full-width at half-maximum	37
G_i	Inhibitory G-protein	12
G_s	Stimulatory G-protein	12
GABA	Gamma-aminobutyric acid	12
GIRK channel	G-protein coupled inward rectifying potassium channel	13
GnRH	Gonadotropin releasing hormone	24
$H_2{}^{15}O$	^{15}O labelled H_2O PET tracer	8
HP-β-CD	Hydroxy-propyl-β-cyclodextrin	22
HPA axis	Hypothalamic-pituitary-adrenal axis	23
HPG	Hypothalamic-pituitary-gonadal axis	23
HVA	4-hydroxy-3-methoxyphenylacetic acid/ homovanillic acid	11
L-DOPA	L-dihydroxphenylalanine	4
LH	Luteinising hormone	24
LTD	Long-term depression	45
MDBF	Multidimensional mood questionnaire	89
MPH	Methylphenidate	75
MS	Magnetic stimulation	52
MT	Motor threshold	10
NE	Norepinephrine	11
NET	Norepinephrine transporter	75

OFC	Orbitofrontal cortex	5
PET	Positron emission tomography	7
PFC	Prefrontal cortex	5
rCBF	Regional cerebral blood flow	8
ROI	Region of interest	39
SD	Standard deviation	37
SEM	Standard error of the mean	24
SHBG	Sex hormone binding globuline	21
SPM	Statistical parametric mapping	39
t_{max}	Time of maximum plasma or saliva concentration	22
TE	Testosterone	4
TH	Tyrosine hydroxylase	11
TMS	Transcranial magnetic stimulation	4
TrpH	Tryptophan hydroxylase	11
VAS	Visual analogue scale	57
VLPFC	Ventrolateral prefrontal cortex	5
VNTR	Variable number tandem repeat	13
VPA	Vaginal pulse amplitude	23
vStr	Ventral striatum	16

Part I

Theoretical Part

Chapter 1
Introduction to the topic

The study of human decision making attempts to understand the fundamental ability to process multiple choice options and to choose an optimal course of action. Decision making refers to the process of selecting one out of several options based on how much reward or punishment each option will bring, on the needs of the decision maker and if learning is involved, on previous experience with the outcomes of the respective options [Doya, 2008]. The recent merging of the two disciplines, neuroscience and economics, has fuelled research on the neurobiological aspects of human decision making. The resulting interdisciplinary research field is termed "neuroeconomics", although it is largely informed by findings from sociology, social psychology, cognitive and neuropsychology. It is therefore often difficult to draw a sharp line between neuroeconomics and social neuroscience, which is a more comprehensive attempt to understand the reciprocal association between social behaviour and neurobiological processes [Cacioppo and Berntson, 2002]. A defining feature of neuroeconomic experiments, including the ones presented in *Chapters 4* and *5*, is the use of monetary incentives to quantify how much an individual subjectively values an outcome of a chosen option. These options are usually presented in the form of paradigms involving one decision maker or many simultaneously interacting decision makers. During individual decision making, the decision maker is confronted with a set of choice options that may include choices between monetary gambles with clearly defined probabilities and outcomes (referred to decision making under risk), choices between monetary gambles of unknown probabilities (decision making under ambiguity) or choices between an immediate, but smaller and a delayed, but larger payoff (intertemporal choice). These choices will only affect the decision maker himself. During social decision making, the decision maker is presented with options that depend also on the decisions of others. Moreover, the decision taken affects other decision makers as well. Such situations are created in the form of simple behavioural tasks derived from experimental economics, in which individuals bargain over money. The standard economic model assumes that individuals behave in a payoff-maximising manner in such situations. However, since fairness, reciprocal, status and other motives are inherent to human social behaviour; these may cause individuals to act in ways that are not profit-maximising. The experimental economics approach allows the assessment of these motives devoid of any social desirability bias, since interactions are set up anonymously. Moreover, by using real monetary incentives, motives can be quantitatively assessed. Finally, deception of the experimental subjects is not allowed for [Hertwig and Ortmann, 2001], *i.e.* the interacting decision makers should all be present in the laboratory, when the decisions are taken. The *Dictator Game* is a well suited paradigm to exemplify the study of social decision making: if a given player A in a dyad receives a certain amount of money of which he can offer a certain amount to a player B, he should offer nothing, if he is profit-maximising. Empirical evidence shows, however, that a significant number of players A offer non-zero amounts to player B, perhaps due to fairness concerns. From this, one can derive that people are willing to sacrifice money because they have non-selfish motives, since it is costly for them to offer non-zero amounts. Naturally, subjects have to believe that the other interaction partner is real, simply because there would otherwise be no reason at all for the players A to offer anything to the players B.

Research into the neurobiology of decision making is largely dominated by correlative studies. Only few studies have used neuromodulatory approaches to investigate a causal relationship between decision making and the underlying neurobiological processes. The three studies presented in this thesis were designed to address some aspects of this gap of knowledge. Experimental modulations on the neurochemical, neuroendocrine and neuroanatomical level will be used to study individual and social decision making, respectively. In particular, a modulation of the dopaminergic (DAergic) system using a single dose of L-dihydroxyphenylalanine (L-DOPA) will be employed to investigate risky decision making. A modulation of the androgen system using a single dose of testosterone (TE) will be used to investigate social bargaining behaviour. Finally, a neurostimulation approach using transcranial magnetic stimulation (TMS) is presented which allows experimental modulation on the anatomical level to investigate aspects of decision making.

Chapter 2

Neuromodulatory approaches to study decision making

2.1 Brain stimulation

Motivation The investigation of the neuroanatomical correlates of risky decision making has received considerable attention so far. A large number of neuroimaging studies revealed brain structures that are activated during risky decision making, including structures related to behavioural control, such as the lateral prefrontal cortex (PFC) (mostly right lateralised) and "reward-related" DAergic brain structures such as the striatum. However, these studies only provide correlative evidence and fail to show a direct causal link between brain structure and function. Investigating patients with focal brain lesions can partially overcome the discrepancy between correlation and causation. Patients who suffer from traumatic injuries of the PFC exhibit profound problems with behavioural control, including problems with self-conduct and in making decisions within the context of their everyday lives [Damasio, 1994]. Moreover, they show an apparent disregard for negative consequences of their actions [Rahman et al., 2001]. In line with these observations are the findings in patients with ventrolateral prefrontal cortex (VLPFC) and orbitofrontal cortex (OFC) lesions who show pronounced risk-seeking behaviour in various gambling tasks, including the *Iowa Gambling Task* and the *Cambridge Gamble Task* [Clark et al., 2003, Manes et al., 2002, Floden et al., 2008]. Little is known, however, about functional compensation following brain damage; although lesions may appear focal, their impact on remote brain regions may be substantial. This prevents us from transferring observations from the lesioned to the healthy brain. Moreover, patients with brain lesions often require anti-convulsive medication, constituting an additional confound. TMS offers a means for overcoming some of the limitations of lesion studies. Its ability to disrupt normal function of human brain transiently makes it a unique tool for studying the causal contribution of different brain areas to human behaviour, including risk taking behaviour. This section offers a short review of the use of TMS to study the role of the dorsolateral prefrontal cortex (DLPFC) in risk taking and outlines the questions that arise from the approach used therein. The study presented in *Chapter 3* was designed to answer some of these questions.

2.1.1 Transcranial magnetic stimulation

TMS is based on the principle of electromagnetic induction and utilises a time-varying magnetic field to induce electrical currents in conducting tissue [Jalinous, 1991]. The magnetic field is generated when electrical energy with a very high current (up to 8000 A) for a duration of approximately 250 μs flows through a wired coil placed over the scalp. The magnetic flux density can reach up to 2.5 T under the coil but decays by the square of the distance to the coil. The magnetic field is oriented perpendicularly to the coil and induces currents which are oriented parallel to the plane of the coil. An obvious advantage of TMS is that the magnetic field passes the skull practically unhindered and can induce electrical currents in the underlying cortex relatively painlessly. These currents are sufficiently large to cause depolarisation of neurons and can thus induce action potentials. This activation can disrupt ongoing processes in neuronal networks. While the application of single pulse TMS is able to disrupt such a process with a high temporal precision (approximately 1 ms), the duration of the disruption is also very limited. The application of temporally ordered repetitive TMS (rTMS) pulses has been shown to cause a more prolonged disruption of brain function ("virtual lesion", see section 3.7.2 on page 51) [Robertson et al., 2003]. In cognitive neuroscience, the approach most frequently used in recent years is to apply a continuous train of low frequency (1 Hz) rTMS over a given brain region for several min *before* performing a given task. This is often referred to as the "off-line" approach and has the advantage that it partially eludes the unspecific effects of concurrent rTMS stimulation [Abler et al., 2005, Pascual-Leone et al., 1998, Robertson et al., 2003].

By applying low frequency rTMS to the right and the left dorsolateral prefrontal cortices, Knoch et al. [2006a] investigated risky decision making "off-line" using the *Cambridge Gamble Task* [Rogers et al., 1999]. Sham stimulation, which produces a click, but no magnetic field, served as a control condition. Subjects stimulated over the right DLPFC were more likely to choose the high-risk prospect and earned significantly less points than those who were either stimulated over the ho-

2.1. Brain stimulation

mologue contralateral site or received sham stimulation. The authors suggest that the risk task primarily involves an active suppression of an option that appears most seductive because of the immediate higher payoffs. Moreover, they suggest that rTMS suppression of the right, but not the left PFC reduced inhibitory control, leading to overly risky decision-making. However, this reasoning only applies if a unilateral stimulation leads to unilateral, and not bilateral neurophysiological "off-line" effects.
Using the same task, two positron emission tomography (PET) studies suggest that risky decision making may recruit ventrolateral rather than dorsal aspects of the PFC [Rogers et al., 1999, Rubinsztein et al., 2001]. Furthermore, the ventrolateral areas (mostly right-lateralised) of the PFC are traditionally implicated in inhibitory control functions [Clark et al., 2003]. It is also possible, however, that stimulation of the DLPFC has indirect effects on the VLPFC via a transsynaptic mechanism. Evidence for this hypothesis comes from studies using retrograde and anterograde tracer techniques showing that Brodmann areas (BA) 45/46 and BA47 are interconnected in the macaque brain [Petrides and Pandya, 1999]. Hence, the indirect stimulation of the VLPFC could have accounted for the subjects' reduced inhibitory control over choosing the risky, but more seductive options in the study by Knoch et al. [2006a].
The combination of neuroimaging techniques such as electroencephalography (EEG), functional magnetic resonance imaging (fMRI) or PET with the "off-line" rTMS protocol offers ways to answer these questions. The general idea underlying this approach is to gain information about whole brain activity over time *after* the application of rTMS to the brain region of interest by comparing it with activity *before* stimulation.
The advantage of EEG in probing such effects is that it provides a direct measure of neuronal activity. It suffers, however, from the relative low spatial resolution and fails to provide information about deeper brain structures such as the basal ganglia. The strength of other neuroimaging methods such as PET and fMRI lies in their ability to obtain localised information about activity throughout the brain. However, fMRI is not ideally suited for repeated, task-independent measurements, since a high-pass filter is used in the data pre-processing stage (typical cut-off frequency: 0.008 Hz) to control for scanner drift and therefore prevents the measurement of absolute blood-flow changes over prolonged time periods. Moreover, the strong magnetic field of the MRI scanner also requires the use of non-ferromagnetic TMS coils.
PET constitutes a good compromise with regard to the desired criteria. Radioac-

tively labelled water ($H_2^{15}O$) is a widely used PET tracer in functional neuroimaging. The tracer is injected intravenously and is distributed with the blood throughout the vascular tree. $H_2^{15}O$ acts as a diffusible tracer, entering the perfused brain tissue, and displaying the distribution of regional cerebral blood flow (rCBF), which has been suggested to reflect presynaptic neuronal activity [Jueptner and Weiller, 1995]. $H_2^{15}O$ has a short half-life of approximately 2 min, allowing a series of injections to be performed every 6 – 10 min. Although it has a relatively low temporal and spatial resolution, this method provides direct and quantitative measures of rCBF. Since these are stable over time, serial, task-independent measurements can be taken. Only a few available studies have examined the effects of low frequency rTMS applied to the PFC using either $H_2^{15}O$–PET or fMRI so far (see Table 2.1). No study has looked at the time-course of rCBF effects following low frequency rTMS of the right DLPFC using the "off-line"-approach.

2.1.2 Summary

Evidence from patient studies, neuroimaging, and an rTMS experiment identified the human right lateral PFC as an important substrate for making adaptive decisions under risk. Low frequency rTMS over the course of several min recently received much interest, as it can create "off-line" effects outlasting the stimulation train in the targeted brain area. However, when applied to the right lateral PFC it is not clear how long these effects last and, in particular, which brain regions remote from the stimulated area are affected as well. No previous study has addressed this issue.

2.1. Brain stimulation

Table 2.1: Studies investigating task-independent neurophysiological effects after low-frequency rTMS applied to the DLPFC of healthy subjects.

Study	Technique	Subjects	Stimulation site & parameters	Signal & brain region Increase	Signal & brain region Decrease	Comments
Ohnishi et al. [2004]	$H_2^{15}O$ PET	seven healthy	R DLPFC, 1 Hz, 100% MT, 100 x eight pulses (intermittently), sham-controlled	L: ventral striatum, ventral PFC (BA45/47); R: medial PFC (BA10)	L: none ; R: none	offline
Kimbrell et al. [2002]	FDG-PET	14 healthy	L DLPFC, 1 Hz, 80% MT, 30 min, sham-controlled	L: angular gyrus, cuneus, occipital gyrus; R: post. insula	L: ACC, striatum, cerebellum, hypothalamus; R: ACC, sup. frontal cortex, cerebellum, hypothalamus, midbrain	online
Speer et al. [2003]	$H_2^{15}O$ PET	ten healthy	L DLPFC, 1 Hz, 80, 90, 100, 110, 120% MT, 75 sec x 5, every 10 min (intermittently)	L: insula, striatum, cerebellum; R: ACC, insula, striatum, cerebellum	L: occipital, precuneus, lingual gyrus; R: occipital, precuneus	Pooled changes in activity from subthreshold and suprathreshold stimulation, no effect, under stim site, intensity dependent decrease in activity in PFC
Nahas et al. [2001]	1.5 T fMRI	five healthy	L DLPFC, 1 Hz, 80, 100, 120% MT, 21 x seven pulses (intermittently)	L: midtemporal lobe, DLPFC (BA46), somatosensory cortex (BA4); R: midtemporal lobe, insula, DLPFC (BA46)	L: none; R: none	Online, pooled changes in activity from subthreshold and suprathreshold stimulation, effect under stim site only at 120% MT but not at 100% MT

2.2 Neuropharmacological modulation

Motivation Interpretations based on neuroimaging data are often subject to the reverse inference problem [Poldrack, 2006]. For example, many neuroimaging experiments report that risky decision making recruits DAergic brain structures. If, for example, the choice of an option associated with a high, but unlikely reward reveals an increased blood-flow in striatum, the activity of which is known to be modulated by DA from studies in animals, this observation does not allow the stringent conclusion that this increased blood-flow reflects an involvement of the DAergic system in risky decision making. Yet again, a distinction between causation and correlation can be made also on the systemic level using patient data. Parkinson's disease patients, who have a dysfunctional DAergic system, receive DAergic medication as part of the treatment strategy to alleviate the prominent motor deficits (see section 2.2.3 on page 16). By experimentally investigating these patients during risk taking tasks before and after medication, a causal relationship was revealed between the modulation of the DAergic system and impulsive betting on the *Cambridge Gamble Task* [Cools et al., 2003]. Findings of such studies have converged on a useful model to understand the role of DA in behavioural control and risk taking. It assumes that the DAergic drug doses necessary to remediate the motor symptoms of Parkinson's disease cause a DAergic "overdose" of relatively unaffected brain regions, such as the ventral frontostriatal circuitry, resulting in poor behavioural control. However, this model still suffers from a lack of generalisability, since DA receptor up regulation might have occurred in distinct parts of the brain due to the general reduction in DAergic neurotransmission in Parkinson's disease patients.

With two exceptions [Hamidovic et al., 2008, Riba et al., 2008], neuropharmacological approaches known to modulate the DAergic system have not been used to investigate risk taking behaviour in healthy humans. If such a systemic approach is used, a clearer picture can be drawn by using additional genetic information. For example, we now know of many DA receptor polymorphisms that determine the efficiency of how these receptors convey neurochemical signals. Genetic association studies have linked these polymorphisms to risk taking proneness. However, no study has yet investigated how a modulation of the DAergic system influences risk taking behaviour conditional on genetic information. The study presented in *Chapter 4* was designed to fill this gap of knowledge, based on the theoretical considerations presented in this section.

2.2.1 Dopaminergic system

Biosynthesis and metabolism of dopamine The neurotransmitter DA is biochemically synthesised from the amino acid L-tyrosine. Circulating L-tyrosine is transported through the blood-brain-barrier (BBB) into the cerebrospinal fluid (CSF) and DAergic neurons by amino acid transporter systems. The enzyme tyrosine hydroxylase (TH) hydroxylates it there to L-DOPA. This is also the rate limiting step in the biosynthesis of DA. The enzyme aromatic L-amino acid decarboxylase (AADC) further converts L-DOPA to DA. This enzyme is present in many types of neurons, including the cytosol of DAergic neurons and in blood plasma. It rapidly metabolises L-DOPA, such that concentration of L-DOPA in blood and in neurons is usually very low under normal conditions (*i.e.* when the AADC is not inhibited pharmacologically) [Elsworth and Roth, 1997]. The use of L-DOPA to elevate DA concentrations thus requires very high doses, unless a decarboxylase inhibitor such as benserazide is used. It is worthwhile to point out that L-DOPA may inhibit tryptophan hydroxylase (TrpH), thereby decreasing the synthesis of the serotonin (5-HT) precursor 5-hydroxy tryptophan (5-HTP) [Naoi et al., 1994]. Thus, L-DOPA administration may well affect the serotonergic system indirectly.

The enzymes monoamino-oxidase (MAO) and aldehyddehydrogenase (ADH) mainly metabolise DA to dihydroxyphenylacetic acid (DOPAC), while the enzyme catechol-O-methyl-transferase (COMT) converts it to homovanillic acid (HVA). DOPAC may be further metabolised into HVA. There are other minor metabolisation pathways which will not be considered here (see Figure 2.1). The concentration of DOPAC in DA-containing brain areas and in CSF is much lower than that of HVA. Removal of HVA and DOPAC from the brain tissue occurs via an active transporter system from CSF into the blood stream [Kopin, 1985]. These metabolites, HVA in particular, could thus potentially serve as peripherally measurable correlates of brain DA turnover [Prockop et al., 1974]. However, DA is also metabolised into the neurotransmitter norepinephrine (NE). This step requires the presence of a specific enzyme, DA-β-hydroxylase (DBH), which is present in sympathetic neurons and in locus coeruleus neurons [Kopin, 1985, Curet et al., 1985]. Therefore, L-DOPA administration may cause an increase in NE neurotransmission in the brain as well. This issue and the fact mentioned above that L-DOPA may inhibit TrpH

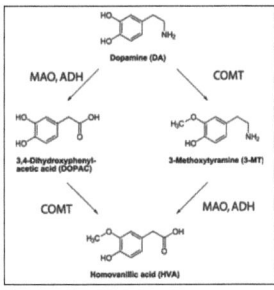

Figure 2.1: Human brain metabolism of DA.

are critical in defining L-DOPA's relative DAergic specificity and will be discussed in section 4.6.4 on page 68.

Dopamine receptors Five DA receptors are known and are all members of the superfamily of seven transmembrane domain G-protein coupled receptors. Based on shared pharmacological features, second messenger coupling, and conserved structural features among individual receptors, they are clustered into D1 and D2-like families of receptors. The D1-like DA receptors consist of the D1 and the D5 receptors. These two receptors share similar pharmacological profiles and are coupled to adenylate cyclase via a stimulatory G-protein (G_s). The D2-like family of DA receptors consists of the D2, D3 and D4 receptors which are coupled to adenylate cyclase via an inhibitory G-protein (G_i) [Bloom et al., 1995]. These two subtypes of DA receptors have differential effects on the formation of cyclic adenosine monophosphate (cAMP) via regulating activity of the adenylate cyclase.

The DA D4 receptor (DRD4) is of particular importance if the current framework, because variants of its gene have been linked to behavioural phenotypes (see section 2.2.1 on page 13) that are potentially relevant for risky decision making. Immunohistochemical studies in the primate brain indicate that the D4 receptor is present in both pyramidal and in higher density on non-pyramidal neurons of the cerebral cortex as well as in the hippocampus [Mrzljak et al., 1996, Lidow et al., 1998]. Most of the non-pyramidal neurons that express the D4 receptor are gamma-aminobutyric acid (GABA) releasing interneurons [Mrzljak et al., 1996]. Activation of D4 receptors reduces GABA-A receptor currents via G_i - mediated reduction of cAMP signalling in rat prefrontal cortical pyramidal neurons [Wang et al., 2002].

Autoradiographic methods are often used to visualise the distribution of specific receptors in human *post-mortem* brains. With respect to the D4 receptor this has been difficult, however, due to a lack of available, selective radioligands. Early studies used subtractive methods which take advantage of the fact that the D4 receptor has a low affinity for C^{11}-raclopride (a selective D2/D3 receptor antagonist) but high affinity to the D2/D3/D4 receptor antagonists H^3-spiperone or H^3-nemonapride [Seeman et al., 1993]. The subtraction of the brain distribution of C^{11}-raclopride binding from H^3-spiperone binding revealed D4 receptor distribution in the PFC and hippocampus. Although the results regarding the presence or absence of the D4 receptor in striatum is somewhat conflicting [Oak et al., 2000], the most selective radioligand H^3–NGD94-1 available did not detect D4 binding sites in striatum of human *post-mortem* brain sections. Binding was observed predominantly in areas of the cerebral cortex, septum, hippocampus, amygdala and hypothalamus [Primus et al., 1997, Lahti et al., 1997].

Dopamine receptor D4 exon III VNTR polymorphism The D4 receptor gene contains a highly polymorphic region within its third exon, also referred to as the DRD4 exon III variable number tandem repeat (VNTR) polymorphism (DRD4 polymorphism). This 48 base-pair polymorphic region encodes a proline-rich protein domain in the third cytoplasmatic loop of the DRD4. The DRD4 polymorphism is an imperfect repeat translated into 16 amino acids found to be present 2-11 times in different alleles of DRD4 [Oldenhof et al., 1998]. The most common alleles in humans are variants with two, four and seven repeats (2R, 4R and 7R, respectively) [van Tol et al., 1992]. The 4R allele is found most frequently (global allele frequency of 64%), followed by the 7R allele (21%) and the 2R allele (8%). High differences occur, however, in frequency distributions among different populations with the 7R allele being virtually absent in Asiatic populations [Chang et al., 1996].
Various attempts have been made to investigate potential differences in the molecular biological properties of the D4 variants. Only the variants which occur most frequently in humans will be mentioned here. It has been hypothesised that the different cytoplasmatic loops might interact differently with downstream G-proteins thereby changing second-messenger signalling efficiency [Lichter et al., 1993]. Accordingly, the 7R variant has been associated with a two-fold diminished potency of DA to inhibit forskolin stimulated cAMP formation compared to the 2R and the 4R variants [Asghari et al., 1995]. Others have shown that the amount of expression of the 7R sequence was lower compared to the 2R and 4R variants [Schoots and Van Tol, 2003]. Moreover, differences in folding efficiency have been shown, with the shorter repeat sequence coding for a more efficiently folded protein and the longer repeat sequence for a less efficiently folded protein [van Craenenbroeck et al., 2005]. In summary, these studies suggest the following order of functional potency of the D4 receptor variants: $7R < 4R = 2R$.
A recent experiment [Wedemeyer et al., 2007] suggested significant differences in electrophysiological responses after DA binding. The three receptor isoforms (2R, 4R and 7R variants) were expressed on a *xenopus laevis* oocyte (egg of African clawed frog) together with a G-protein coupled inward rectifying K^+ channel (GIRK). Previous evidence showed that the D4 receptor readily couples to GIRK channels [Werner et al., 1996]. The effective DA concentration necessary to induce GIRK mediated K^+ currents was approximately five-fold lower for the 2R and the 7R receptor variants compared to the 4R variant. This study is important because it suggests a different order of functional potency of these variants: $7R = 2R > 4R$.

DRD4 exon III VNTR polymorphism and human behaviour An increasing amount of studies, however, link the single DRD4 exon III VNTR polymorphism to a number of human traits and behaviours which are relevant in the context of risk taking. When comparing different variants of a given allele contributing to behaviour, it has to be kept in mind that the comparison of genotypes and their behavioural correlates is always relative. The rationales for forming groups according to genotypes can comprise arguments based on functional potency of the different receptor variants (see above), but it can also entail evolutionary aspects. For example, it has been suggested that the 7R allele arose from the 4R allele as a rare mutation event some 40'000 y ago, and has been under positive selection ever since [Wang et al., 2004]. This suggests that the 4R variant could be used as a "reference" when comparing it with carriers of the 7R variant. The most often used approach in the literature is either the comparison of the most common with a specific genotype (*e.g.*, 4/4 vs 4/7) or the comparison of subjects who carry at least one "special" allele (*e.g.* the 7R allele) with those who do not carry the allele. In most studies, the 2R variant is neglected, which is mostly due to the fact that its frequency is considerably lower than that of the 4R and the 7R variants. It should be emphasised that the attempt to link one single gene to one single behaviour is an oversimplification of complex neurobiological processes, which most consider untenable (see also section 4.6.6 on page 70).

Ebstein et al. [1996] initiated research into the behavioural phenotypes associated with the DRD4 exon III polymorphism. They reported that the 7R variant carriers have higher scores on the sensation-seeking dimension of Cloninger's tridimensional personality questionnaire [Cloninger et al., 1991], which has been widely used in genetic association studies. However, this finding appears to be somewhat inconsistent and has spurred a dispute in the literature. It has been suggested, for example, that it may not be the DRD4 genotype *per se*, but rather an interaction with substance use or abuse associated with novelty-seeking [Lusher et al., 2001, Kluger et al., 2002]. There is indeed evidence that links this polymorphism with increased odds for substance addiction [Comings et al., 1999]. The issue remains similarly inconclusive, however, since other studies also failed to find such effects [Lusher et al., 2001]. It is worthwhile to mention, however, that subjects who carry the 7R variant of the receptor seem to face an increased likelihood of suffering from pathological gambling [Perez de Castro et al., 1997]. The most consistent finding is the association of the 7R variant with attention deficit hyperactivity disorder (ADHD), a childhood-onset psychiatric disorder whose cardinal symptoms are inattention, hyperactivity, and impulsivity [Faraone et al., 2001, Li et al., 2006]. ADHD

2.2. Neuropharmacological modulation

affects an estimated 3% of elementary school children. As in all association studies, one cannot assume that the presence of the 7R allele is neither necessary nor sufficient to "cause" ADHD. Interestingly however, it was found that *among* children with ADHD, carriers of the 7R allele differed significantly from the group without this allele in that they were faster and less accurate in the *Matching Familiar Figures Test*, suggesting higher impulsivity in these children [Langley et al., 2004]. A similar finding was observed in a sample of healthy adults showing that 7R carriers have a significantly longer reaction time on the *Stop Signal Task* (compared to carriers without the 7R allele), suggesting poor inhibitory control in these subjects [Congdon et al., 2008].

2.2.2 Pharmacogenetics and behaviour

The term "pharmacogenetics" refers to the study of the hereditary basis for differences in drug responses. While a wealth of pharmacogenetic research has focused on individuals' genetic susceptibility to adverse drug reactions [Pirmohamed, 2001, Pirmohamed and Park, 2001] and how polymorphisms and mutations in neurotransmitter receptors can alter functional activity and pharmacological profiles [Wong et al., 2000], only little evidence is available that links receptor gene variants to drug responses in terms of human behaviour. With respect to the serotonergic system, a number of studies investigated the interaction of tryptophan depletion, which is an way to lower 5-HT transmission in the CNS, with the serotonin-transporter polymorphism (5HTTPP) on object choice [Blair et al., 2008], recognition of fear facial expressions [Marsh et al., 2006], passive avoidance and response reversal instrumental learning performance [Finger et al., 2007], emotional processing, memory and attention [Roiser et al., 2007] and performance on a cued reinforcement reaction time task [Roiser et al., 2006]. Only one study is presently available with respect to the DAergic system. This study used cabergoline, a fairly selective D2 receptor agonist, to investigate reversal learning performance conditional on the *Taq*1A DA D2 receptor polymorphism (DRD2 polymorphism) . Compared with placebo, cabergoline administration made A1+ allele carriers take significantly longer to reach learning criteria, but made A1- allele carriers learn faster [Cohen et al., 2007]. With respect to the DRD4 polymorphism, no studies are available that investigated pharmacogenetic effects on behaviour.

2.2.3 Pathological gambling in Parkinson's disease patients

Parkinson's disease is a neurodegenerative disease characterised by a progressive loss of DAergic neurons in the nigrostriatal and, to a lesser extent, in the mesocorticolimbic system. In early Parkinson's disease, DA depletion is restricted to the putamen and the dorsal caudate nucleus, and later progresses to the more ventral parts of the striatum and the mesocorticolimbic DAergic system [Kish et al., 1988]. Administering L-DOPA is efficient for treating the motor symptoms, however, the effect on cognitive functions seems to be two-fold: medication ameliorates deficits on set-shifting, associated with dorsal striatal-DLPFC circuitry [Sohn et al., 2000], while it impairs performance on probabilistic reversal learning, associated with ventral fronto-striatal circuitry [Cools et al., 2002]. Based on this and previous work [Gotham et al., 1986, Swainson et al., 2000], the hypothesis was formulated that L-DOPA normalises DA levels in severely depleted areas in the Parkinsonian brain, such as the dorsal striatum and its connections to the DLPFC, while "overdosing" the relatively intact ventral striatum (vStr) and its connections to the ventral PFC [Cools et al., 2003]. This "overdose" hypothesis is based on evidence suggesting that there is an optimal amount of DA receptor stimulation, meaning that too little or too much stimulation of DA receptors decreases several performance and neural activity measures ("inverted-U" relationship) [Williams and Goldmanrakic, 1995, Vijayraghavan et al., 2007]. .

Thus, a relative DA "overdose" of the ventral frontostriatal circuitry might explain a diminished performance during reversal learning tasks; the poorer performance reflects impaired impulse control [Dias et al., 1996]. Following this line of reasoning, it was hypothesised that L-DOPA administration causes impulse control deficits in early stage Parkinson's disease patients. The procedure most commonly employed to assess the neuropsychological effects of L-DOPA in Parkinson's disease patients is the controlled L-DOPA withdrawal procedure. It requires patients to abstain from their L-DOPA for a period of approximately 15 h prior to the neuropsychological assessment. Performance in this "off-state" state is compared with that in a separate testing session during which patients take their medication as usual, the "on-state" [Cools et al., 2006]. This procedure showed that patients who were in the "on-state" exhibited more impulsive betting strategies in the *Cambridge Gamble Task*, relative to the "off-state" [Cools et al., 2003]. Figure 2.2 depicts an illustration of the "overdose"-model, based on the hypothesis initially put forward by Swainson et al. [2000] and extended by the current state of knowledge [Cools et al., 2003, 2006, Cools, 2008]. Consistent with the finding of a generally decreased impulse control in medicated early-stage Parkinson's disease patients is the observation of

2.2. Neuropharmacological modulation

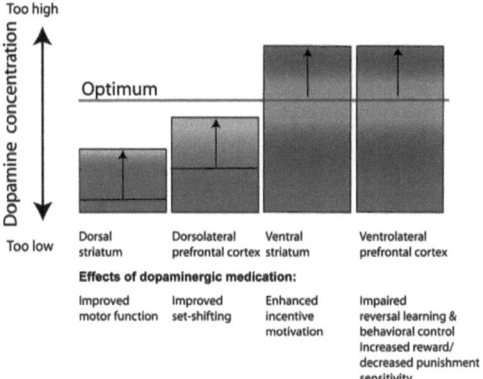

Figure 2.2: The DA "overdose" hypothesis applied to cognitive functions within dorsal and ventral frontostriatal circuitry. DA depletion severe enough to produce functional deficits may be present in all regions of the putamen and only in the most dorsal, rostral aspect of the head of the caudate nucleus thereby affecting only the motor system and the dorsolateral prefrontal loops. DAergic medication results in beneficial effects on motor control and set-shifting in these loops; it may, however increase the amount of DAergic activity above the optimal level in the less affected ventromedial head and tail of the caudate nucleus (parts of the VLPFC respectively), resulting in impaired reversal learning, decreased behavioural control, and increased reward/ decreased punishment sensitivity. The arrows indicate the potential direction of effects of a particular dose of DAergic medication on levels of overall DAergic activity and on task performance. Adapted from Swainson et al. [2000].

pathological gambling in these patients. Pathological gambling is classified as an impulse control disorder and defined as a failure to resist gambling impulses despite severe personal, familial, and financial losses [APA, 1995]. While the lifetime prevalence of pathological gambling in the North American general population is 1.6%, it was reported to lie between 3% and 8% in Parkinson's disease patients using medication [Voon et al., 2007a]. Molina et al. [2000] investigated a sample of 250 patients receiving L-DOPA and identified twelve who had problems with gambling. Importantly, ten started gambling after the onset of L-DOPA treatment, suggesting a causal role of DAergic drug treatment in the aetiology of the gambling disorder.

2.2.4 Summary

In healthy humans, relatively few studies are available that examined the role of DA in risky decision making from a pharmacological perspective. Showing that a relatively coarse manipulation of the DAergic system can alter risky decision making would be an initial step in bridging this gap. The DA precursor L-DOPA is a useful substance for achieving this for two reasons: first, it increases the presynaptic availability of DA without having direct effects on specific subtypes of receptors. Second, evidence from studies of Parkinson's disease patients suggests that L-DOPA treatment might be associated with decreased impulse control and pathological gambling. Thus, findings in these patients can serve as a model for investigating healthy humans in a placebo-controlled L-DOPA administration study. To provide more specificity, additional genetic information at the receptor level can be introduced. The D4 receptor seems to be a promising candidate, given its reported association with impulsivity and impulse control related disorders, including ADHD and pathological gambling. Such a pharmacogenetic approach allows investigating the influence of L-DOPA on risk taking behaviour in subpopulations identified through the DRD4 polymorphism, whereby the common group (4R allele carriers) may acts as a control group for the 7R allele carriers. So far, no study has used this approach in the domain of risky decision making in humans.

2.3 Neuroendocrine modulation

Motivation While the use of modulatory approaches to investigate the neuroendocrinological aspects of social decision making has just recently begun [Kosfeld et al., 2005, Baumgartner et al., 2008], neuroendocrine "biomarkers" such as salivary and serum measures of sex hormones have long been used to predict human social behaviour. TE, which is perhaps the best known sex hormone, has received paramount attention. As early as the seventies, [Ehrenkranz et al., 1974] reported that serum concentrations of TE is positively related to dominant social behaviour in male prisoners. Many experiments followed and the possibility of detecting hormones in saliva [Landman et al., 1976] set the stage for large scale field experiments investigating the neuroendocrine correlates of human social behaviour. This work has posed a major challenge for sociologists, because it represented a shift away from the classical sociological injunction that social behaviour can only be explained by social facts [Udry et al., 1995]. Those who agreed with the idea that biological factors may also influence our social behaviour have defined a new inter-

2.3. Neuroendocrine modulation

disciplinary research field, termed "biosociology". Two important models emerged from his field: *the basal model*, which assumes that endogenous TE levels can be thought of as a trait, whereby individual differences in basal TE cause variation in dominance (*i.e.* enhancing of one's status over that of other people) and the *reciprocal model*, which assumes that certain social situations (such as dominance disputes and competition) cause TE levels to change, and that these changes in TE then feed back to reinforce or discourage further behaviours which led to the TE change in the first place [Mazur and Booth, 1998]. The measurement of endogenous TE levels obviously does not provide evidence that TE actually causes the behaviour in question. The reciprocal model suggests particular caution in interpreting correlative data gained from field studies. A well suited example for describing this issue is the following study: Coates and Herbert [2008] investigated a sample of stock-market traders and their salivary TE levels. They reported that a trader's morning TE level was positively related with his day's profitability on the stock market. However, according to the reciprocal model, it might well be the case that a successful trader experienced a TE surge due to his profitable trading behaviour in the morning. Thus, morning trading performance would perhaps have been a better predictor of a trader's day's profitability. Morning TE levels would therefore reflect a subsidiary variable, rather than a good predictor. By using economic social interaction paradigms, which quantify social decision making behaviour in the context of a well controlled experimental environment, many limitations of these field studies can be overcome. Moreover, the combination of placebo-controlled TE administration using such paradigms offers insight into the causal relationship between TE and social decision making behaviour. In this section, a general overview of the pharmacological properties of TE and its behavioural effects in animals and humans will be given. The study presented in *Chapter 5* resulted from the considerations herein.

2.3.1 The androgen system

Biosynthesis of testosterone TE is synthesised from cholesterol in five basic enzymatic steps. First, cholesterol is converted to pregnenolone. This is the rate-limiting step in the synthesis of all steroid hormones. The conversion encompasses three sub steps - C20-hydroxylation, C22-hydroxylation, and cleavage of the C20-C22 bond - to produce pregnenolone and isocaproic acid. These three sub steps are mediated by a single mitochondrial cytochrome [$P450_{scc}$, Chung et al., 1986]. In a second step, pregnenolone is hydroxylated at the C17 position by the steroid-17-hydroxylase (cytochrome $P450_{c17}$) to form 17-hydroxy-pregnenolone. A third enzymatic step involving a C17/C20 lyase (cytochrome $P450_{c17}$) yields dihydroepiandrosterone (DHEA). The fourth and fifth metabolic steps include reduction to androstenedione (by the 17-β-hydroxysteroid dehydrogenase [17-β-HSD]) and ultimately the conversion to TE by the 17-β-HSD. TE is the main androgen in the human body and is characterised by an oxygen group at position C3, a hydroxy group at position C17 and a double bond in position C4 [Voet et al., 1992, Nieschlag, 2006]. The following paragraph briefly describes the sources of androgens in females, since the experiment described in *Chapter 5* was conducted with female subjects exclusively. TE is secreted by the adrenal zona fasciculata (25%) and the ovarian stroma (25%), the remaining 50% are produced from circulating androgens such as DHEA. DHEA is primarily an adrenal product, regulated by the adrenocorticotropic hormone (ACTH) and acts as a precursor for the peripheral synthesis of more potent androgens such as TE and dihydrotestosterone (DHT) [Davis and Burger, 2003]. Daily production rate of TE is in the order of 0.1 − 0.4 mg and circulating levels are in the range of 0.2 − 0.7 ng/ml (0.6 − 2.5 nmol/l). TE is at its lowest concentrations in the early follicular phase of the cycle and rises to a mid-cycle peak [Abraham, 1974]. The following luteal phase concentrations are higher than those in the early follicular phase. Hormone assays have indicated that TE shows circadian variation, peak levels being seen in the early morning hours [Davis and Burger, 2003].

Metabolism TE is metabolised both into active and inactive metabolites. The formation of the inactive metabolites involves hydroxylation at the C6, C7, C15, C16 positions, glucuronidation at the C3 or C17 position and subsequent excretion of these metabolites via the urinary pathway. Androsteron and etiocholanone are the most abundant urinary androgen metabolites [Nieschlag, 2006] and play an important role in detecting abuse of anabolic steroids in urine by athletes [Catlin et al., 1997]. TE is, however, also metabolised into the highly neuroactive steroids DHT and 17β-estradiol (E2). E2 results from an aromatisation of TE at the C4 position by the enzyme aromatase; DHT results from reduction of TE via the 5α-reductase. Since many of TE's actions are assumed to result from its conversion to these neuroactive metabolites, it has also been referred to as a *prohormone* (see section 5.5.3 on page 97).

Transport and blood-brain barrier permeability By virtue of its lipophilicity, TE diffuses easily through cell membranes including the capillary walls of the BBB without the need of an active transporter mechanism (William M. Pardridge, *personal communication*). A significant proportion of hormones is bound to globu-

2.3. Neuroendocrine modulation

lins present in serum. The globulins are specific for classes of hormones; the sex hormone binding globulin (SHBG) binds TE and E2 and occurs in such species as primates but not rodents [Corvol and Bardin, 1973]. The hormone fraction in plasma available for transport into brain is inversely related to the amount of SHBG present in the circulation [Pardridge and Mietus, 1979].

Pharmacodynamics   Both TE and DHT bind to the androgen receptor (AR). Although it was initially assumed that steroids exert their effects uniquely through a *genomic* pathway via intracellularly located receptors, it is now recognised that they may also act through a *non-genomic* pathway via membrane bound receptors [for a review, see Simoncini and Genazzani, 2003]. The genomic pathway involves diffusion of the steroid through the cell membrane, binding of the hormone to the AR, separation of the receptor from cytoplasmic chaperone proteins (hsp-90), translocation of the receptor from the cytosol into the nucleus and dimerisation of the receptor. This dimer binds to specific hormone-responsive elements on the desoxynucleic acid (DNA) resulting in down- or up regulation of transcription of certain genes [Voet et al., 1992]. This mode of action is considered to be slow, ranging from hours to days. The non-genomic pathway does not depend on gene transcription or protein synthesis and involves steroid-induced modulation of cell membrane-bound regulatory proteins coupled to ion-channels [Simoncini and Genazzani, 2003].

DHT is also a classical androgen binding exclusively to the AR. It has however, a fourfold higher affinity to the receptor than TE [Grino et al., 1990]. Moreover, it exhibits a five-fold slower dissociation rate from the receptor, compared to TE. As a consequence, substantially lower concentrations of DHT are necessary to activate cellular processes [Grino et al., 1990]. E2 activates the estrogen receptor type alpha (ER-α) and type beta (ER-β) in several tissues including different areas of the brain [Couse et al., 1999]. The conversion of TE to E2 gives rise to a number of questions in interpreting results from TE modulation experiments. These will be discussed in section 5.5.3 on page 97.

Testosterone preparations   A number of TE preparations (injectables, oral and sublingual formulations and gels) are available allowing the experimental manipulation of TE levels in humans to investigate causality in social decision making behaviour. In order to have good experimental control, TE administration and behavioural testing should be performed in the same experimental session. This ensures that no experiences outside the laboratory (perhaps influenced by TE administration) confound social decision making behaviour in the laboratory. Therefore, the duration until the maximum blood concentration is achieved after TE administration (t_{max}) is an important parameter. The following paragraphs briefly describe the pharmacokinetic parameters of some of the available compounds as well as their advantages and limitations.

Injectable forms of testosterone The injectable TE preparations available have important clinical importance in the treatment of male hypogonadism [Behre et al., 1999]. Most of them are also illicitly used by athletes to increase muscle mass. The intramuscular injection of TE-esters is the most widely used approach for TE substitution therapy of male hypogonadism. For these purposes, chemical esterification of TE has to be performed, since unmodified TE has a half-life of only 10 min and would thus have to be injected very frequently. Esterification at position C17 of the molecule prolongs the half-life in proportion to the length of the added side-chain. These side-chains usually derive from propionic acid, enanthic acid, cypionic acid or undecanoic acid, resulting in TE-ester half-lives of 0.8, 4.5, 29.5 and 33.9 d, respectively [Nieschlag, 2006]. For a number of reasons, these preparations are all not favourable for investigating decision making in humans. First, even the fastest acting preparation, TE-propionate, does not reach t_{max} until 14 h after administration [Nieschlag, 2006]. Second, subjects who are afraid of injections might experience stress and this may itself lead to altered TE secretion from the adrenal gland (see page 25). Third, the time course of neurophysiological effects in the central nervous system (CNS) is not known. A sublingual application of TE in female subjects can overcome these limitations.

Sublingual administration From a pharmacological viewpoint, the resorption of TE through the oral mucosa is advantageous, since it leads to a rapid rise in systemic TE concentrations but also avoids the pronounced intestinal and hepatic first pass metabolism usually observed if ingested orally. Moreover, it is non-invasive. However, since TE is hydrophobic, it does not dissolve in saliva and it is therefore difficult to bring the molecule into close contact with the cell membranes of the oral mucosa. The use of hydroxy-propyl-β-cyclodextrin (HP-β-CD) [Figure 2.3 (**A**)] inclusion complexes as a carrier system can overcome this obstacle. Cyclodextrins are cyclic oligosaccharides consisting of a number of dextrose molecules. All secondary hydroxyl groups are located on one edge of the molecule, while the primary hydroxyl groups are located on the other edge. The internal cavity of HP-β-CD is relatively hydrophobic, and thus, lipophilic guest molecules such as TE reside partially within the ring cavity of the cyclodextrin without being covalently bound to

2.3. Neuroendocrine modulation

the host molecule. In solution with saliva, the cyclodextrin solubilises the otherwise insoluble TE, and the lipophilic TE molecules are absorbed by the oral mucosa and eventually enter the systemic circulation [Hirayama and Uekama, 1999]. Stuenkel et al. [1991] showed that the sublingual administration of 2.5 mg and 5 mg TE complexed with HP-β-CD to hypogonadal males leads to a rapid increase in serum TE concentrations [Figure 2.3 (**B**)] and Tuiten et al. [2000] reported similar pharmacokinetics after the application of 0.5 mg of sublingual TE to healthy female subjects [Figure 2.3 (**C**)]. So far, this is the only study that has investigated the time-course of neurophysiological effects after a single-dose of TE in healthy humans [Tuiten et al., 2000]. The authors reported a significant increase in vaginal pulse amplitude (VPA, a measure reflecting vaginal blood-flow and sexual arousal) in response to the presentation of erotic movie clips after about 4 h. This effect was absent when movies with a neutral content were presented, suggesting that the effects on the VPA was not related to unspecific vasodilatatory effects of TE [Figure 2.3 (**D**)]. The VPA seems to be the only physiological response known to possess a non-habitual nature, thus allowing multiple measures throughout the day. In summary, this study provides evidence that neurophysiological effects following a single sublingual administration of 0.5 mg TE peak 2.5 h after that TE levels in the blood have already returned to baseline [Tuiten et al., 2000]. It was hypothesised that this time lag is due to the genomic way of action of TE.

2.3.2 Neuroendocrinology

The two neuroendocrine regulatory systems, the hypothalamic-pituitary-gonadal axis (HPG axis) and the hypothalamic-pituitary-adrenal axis (HPA axis), are interdependent systems each affecting one another. The HPA axis is a system which is activated during physiological (infections, injuries) as well as psychological stress (as part of the fight-or-flight response) [Hellhammer, 2008]. It triggers the release of three key hormones (corticotropin-releasing hormone [CRH], adrenocorticotropic hormone [ACTH] and, in humans, cortisol [CORT]). Stress provokes the release of CRH from the hypothalamus into the anterior pituitary via the portal vein. Upon activation of CRH receptors, ACTH is released into the general circulation. ACTH triggers the biosynthesis and release of CORT from the adrenal cortex into the bloodstream. The HPA axis is controlled via a negative feedback system in which the end product, CORT, inhibits the production of the initiation substance, CRH. In addition, CORT inhibits ACTH secretion [Miller and O'Callaghan, 2002, Birbaumer and Schmidt, 2006].
The HPG-axis regulates development and reproductive function of the gonads. More-

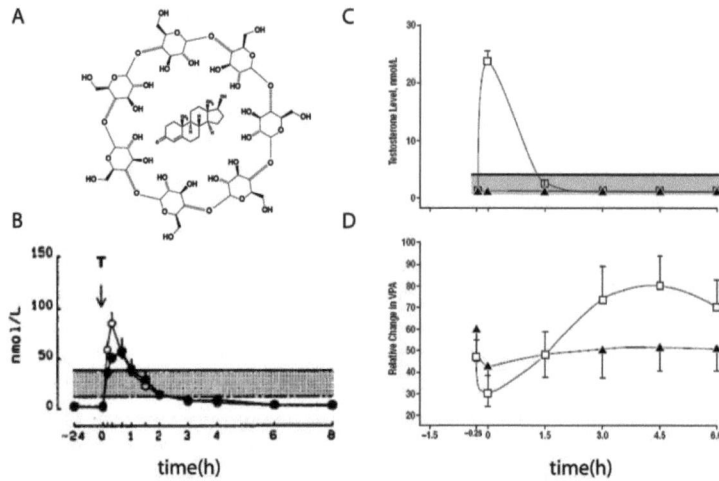

Figure 2.3: (A) The basic structure of the TE- hydroxy-propyl-β-cyclodextrin inclusion complex, which can be administered sublingually. (B) Pharmacokinetics of serum TE after the administration of a single dose of 2.5 mg (○) and 5.0 mg (•) of sublingual TE to five hypogonadal men. The shaded area indicates the normal physiological range of TE levels in males. (C) Pharmacokinetics of serum TE after administration of a single dose of 0.5 mg of sublingual TE (□) or placebo (▲) to eight healthy females. (D) Average relative increase in vaginal pulse amplitude (VPA) induced by erotic film excerpts viewed at six consecutive times during placebo (▲) and TE (□) treatment in eight healthy females. Error bars indicate SEM.

over, it controls sex hormone production via hormone-dependent feedback loops. This feedback loop consists of the key hormones gonadotropin-releasing-hormone (GnRH), luteinising-hormone (LH), follicle-stimulating hormone (FSH) and the male (androgens) and female sex hormones (estrogens and gestagens). GnRH is released from the hypothalamus in a pulsatile fashion. These pulses will only stimulate the release of LH and FSH from the anterior pituitary into the blood-stream if they are generated in a regular fashion. In the female ovaries, FSH stimulates the growth of immature follicles to maturation. In male testes, FSH stimulates spermatogenesis. LH regulates the biosynthesis and secretion of androgens in males. TE is secreted into the blood-stream in spurts, and measured levels can change considerably within a few min. In females, LH regulates the biosynthesis and secretion of

2.3. Neuroendocrine modulation

both androgens and estrogens. Moreover, LH triggers ovulation which releases the egg from the follicle and initiates the conversion of the residual follicle into a corpus luteum that, in turn, produces progesterone [Birbaumer and Schmidt, 2006].
Chemical castration takes advantage of the fact that GnRH *pulsatility* is necessary for LH and FSH secretion. Thus, by applying either a GnRH agonist or antagonist with a long half-life, both of which continuously occupy GnRH receptors, the secretion of the gonadotropins LH and FSH can be suppressed [Nieschlag, 2006]. A temporary chemical castration and subsequent placebo-controlled administration of TE would be the state-of-the-art model for investigating the causal role of TE in human decision making behaviour. Although this method is clearly superior to a simple placebo-controlled administration of TE, it was not considered suitable for the study that will be presented in *Chapter 5* for ethical reasons.

Stress as a modulator of testosterone secretion Stress can influence TE at the level of the hypothalamus, pituitary gland, and adrenal cortex. Since DHEA, which is mainly a product from the adrenal cortex regulated by ACTH, is the source for up to 50% of the female production of TE, increasing DHEA levels will lead to changes in TE levels [Burger and Davis, 2002, see also section 2.3.1 on page 20]. Thus, acute stress, which leads to increased levels of ACTH, might cause increased TE levels in females. On the other hand, it has been suggested that prolonged stress may act at the level of the pituitary and hypothalamus to suppress LH and GnRH pulsatility [Tilbrook et al., 2000] which could lead to lowered TE levels secreted from the ovaries.

2.3.3 Behavioural effects of testosterone

The effects of TE in adults depend on the interaction of long-term organisational and short-term activational effects [Mazur and Booth, 1998]. The organisational effects occur around birth. During fetal and neonatal life, relatively higher concentrations of TE (in males versus females) are thought to influence brain development by defeminising the brain into a relatively male-like configuration. Studies in rodents and primates have shown that the hypothalamus, the hippocampus, the preoptic-septal region and the limbic system are important target areas for sex steroid action during development [Mcewen, 1992, Collaer and Hines, 1995, Christiansen, 2001]. These brain structures are then thought to be activated later in life, when TE concentrations rise (*e.g.* due to aggressive and non-aggressive battles over status). In the adult male and female brain, highest concentrations of TE are found in the hypothalamus, preoptic area, and substantia nigra as radioimmunoassay of *post-mortem* brains revealed [Bixo et al., 1995].

As it is the case with many neuroactive substances, TE does not cause behavioural changes *per se*; it rather alters the probability that a particular behaviour will occur in the presence of a particular stimulus. For example, if TE levels are within or above the physiological range, the hormones action on hypothalamic regions allows normal sexual interest in males [Christiansen, 2001] and females [Davis and Tran, 2001]. If TE levels are below a certain limit, libido is markedly impaired.

Aggression in rodents The activational effects of TE have been shown in many rodent experiments investigating aggression [*e.g.* Beeman, 1947, Edwards, 1969, Lumia et al., 1994, Melloni et al., 1997]. When caged together, mice usually establish social hierarchies based on dominance-subordination relationships. Such hierarchy formation happens to be established aggressively, sometimes resulting in severe injuries or death of these animals. One of the first comprehensive experiments that investigated the role of TE in aggression in rodents was performed by Beeman [1947]. Aggressive behaviour was assessed in groups of normal (n = 20) and castrated mice (n = 48). They were staged in a neutral cage, which was divided into two equal sections by a partition that could be readily raised. To investigate aggressive behaviour the partition was raised and fighting was observed. Strikingly, *none* of the castrated mice showed any form of aggressive behaviour, while *all* normal mice fought. In a second stage of the experiment, a subset of castrated mice received either a TE propionate (15 mg, n = 25) or dextrose (n = 15) implant. Each of the TE treated mice, but none of those with the dextrose implant, behaved aggressively. This aggression was similar as in normal mice suggesting that TE

2.3. Neuroendocrine modulation

plays a causal role in maintaining the ability to behave aggressively in combat. The organisational effects of TE are illustrated by an experiment performed by Edwards [1969], where the influence of postnatal TE administration on aggressive behaviour in male and female mice that were previously castrated was investigated. The experiment can be summarised in the following way: 1 d after birth, a group of males and a group of females were injected with a vehicle (oil). Another group of females received 0.5 mg of TE 1 d after birth. Yet another group of females received oil 1 d after birth and 0.5 mg of TE 10 d after birth. All mice were castrated 30 d after birth. After 60 d, they were given injections of various doses of TE (oil [sham], 10, 20, 50, 100 & 500 µg). They were then tested in a resident intruder paradigm. A dose-dependent fighting behaviour after pairing was observed, which was highest and identical in males treated with oil and females treated with 0.5 mg of TE 1 d after birth, somewhat lower in females treated with 0.5 mg of TE 10 d after birth and lowest in females treated with oil (Figure 2.4).

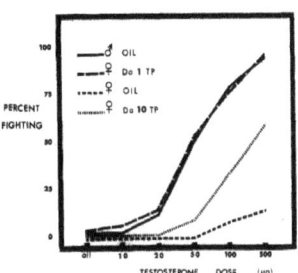

Figure 2.4: The percent of the total number of gonadectomised adult pairs in each group fighting (y-axis) at each dose level of TE (x-axis). Figure taken from Edwards [1969].

These results suggest that there seems to be a critical period for the androgen influenced organisation of the CNS to allow aggression. This period in the development of the mouse may be characterised as a period of time during which endogenous or exogenous TE stimulation will enhance adult sensitivity to androgens with respect to the tendency for aggression. However, it has to be noted that later experiments suggested that E2 is the agent that causes these organisational effects.

2.3.4 Social behaviour in humans

Most studies that investigate the relationship between TE and social behaviour are correlative, meaning that endogenous TE levels are measured in saliva or serum and correlated with a behavioural measure or questionnaire scores. Most of these correlative studies are based on an important premise, according to which TE levels can be thought of as a trait, whereby individual differences in basal TE cause variation in social behaviours. This has been referred to as the *basal model*. In support of this model is evidence that basal TE levels are relatively temporally stable across 5 d [Sellers et al., 2007], 8 wk [Dabbs, 1990], or even 1 y [Granger et al., 2004]. Moreover, there is evidence from twin studies showing that basal TE levels are partly heritable [Harris et al., 1998]. Taken together, these findings support the basal model and suggest that basal TE can be thought of as an individual difference variable that explains distinct domains of our social behaviour.

Anti-social behaviour Putatively driven by the scientific findings of TE induced aggression in rodents and the case reports describing steroid induced rage, a number of studies sought to establish a link between TE and violent and anti-social behaviour in humans. Several studies aimed at establishing such a relationship with prison inmates. Generally, a positive relationship between basal TE levels and past crime severity could be established [Dabbs et al., 1995, Dabbs and Hargrove, 1997]. However, prison inmates constitute a subpopulation with potential confounding pre-existing personality traits such as *e.g.* psychopathy and impulsivity. A more comprehensive study was performed by [Dabbs, 1990], in which a sample of 4462 U.S. military veterans was investigated. In this study, subjects who ranged at the top 10% of circulating TE levels were reported to have an increased likelihood of having committed anti-social activities since being 18 years old, including assaultive marital or relationship problems, negligence toward children, job trouble, trouble with debts, traffic offenses, non-traffic arrests, lying, violence, and vagrancy. The authors acknowledged that the effects in the study are small and that only the extreme levels of TE seemed to account for appreciable variance [Dabbs, 1990].

Many researchers in the field of TE research, however, view anti-social behaviour rather as a form of dominance behaviour that occurs in settings where authority figures require behaviour to conform closely to rigid standards and rules. This may occur in schools, prisons, or in the military [Booth et al., 2006]. Individuals who are predisposed to dominant behaviour but hold subordinate positions in settings such as prisons or in the military are likely to break the rules in order to prevail over the constraining environment [Booth et al., 2006].

Dominance, status and leadership In their biosociological review, Mazur and Booth [1998] argue that TE's role in social behaviour is mainly to assert an individual's dominance and status. The main aim of their paper was to dissociate the link between TE induced aggressive dominance behaviour, which is frequently observed in rodents, from a link between TE and non-aggressive dominance behaviour, which is more often observed in non-human primates and humans.

2.3. Neuroendocrine modulation

Dominance is defined as behaviours with the intent to gain or maintain high status [Mazur and Booth, 1998]. Individuals with a high status have unrestricted access to resources and can influence others in the group. Low status individuals have little influence and are constrained in their choices [Mazur, 2005]. The hypothesis that TE is related to status receives support from a number of primate studies, in which it has been shown that endogenous TE levels and the position in the status hierarchy are positively correlated [Rose et al., 1971]. Importantly, the relationship between TE and status tends to emerge most strongly during periods of social instability [Muller and Wrangham, 2004]. In wild baboons for example, TE levels predicted status-related behaviours only after the alpha male had been crippled in fights and the status hierarchy was destabilised. When the hierarchy was stable, however, TE and behaviour were unrelated [Sapolsky, 1991].

The association between TE and dominance has also been extended to humans. For instance, people with high basal TE tend to be more socially dominant and value being in a high status position more highly than individuals with low basal TE [Cashdan, 1995, Grant and France, 2001, Josephs et al., 2003, 2006, Newman et al., 2005, Sellers et al., 2007]. An approach which has often been used to investigate status effects in humans is to randomly assign individuals to victory (high status) and defeat (low status) in competitive social interactions by rigging the outcome of the competitions. These studies showed that individuals with high endogenous TE levels function better in high status positions than in low status ones. Specifically, high TE individuals paid more attention to status cues, became dysphoric, and performed poorly on complex cognitive tasks after a defeat, but paid less attention to status cues, showed no evidence of dysphoria, and performed well on complex cognitive tasks after victory [*e.g.* Josephs et al., 2003, 2006, Newman et al., 2005]. Taken together, these studies suggests that humans with high TE levels experience pleasure and adaptive functioning (*e.g.*, good cognitive performance) when they achieve high status. When they fail to achieve high status, however, individuals high in TE experience dysphoria and maladaptive functioning (*e.g.*, poor cognitive performance).

The main body of research examining TE and dominance has been conducted in men [Mazur and Booth, 1998, Grant and France, 2001]. A small, but growing literature suggests, however, that basal TE may also explain status seeking behaviours in women. For example, women with high basal TE tend to have dominant personalities [Dabbs and Hargrove, 1997, Dabbs et al., 1988] and occupy high socioeconomic status positions such as being a student, managerial, or technical worker [Purifoy and Koopmans, 1979]. Moreover, female adolescents with relatively high TE levels more often chose the words "enterprising", "initiative", "original", and "dominant" to describe themselves in an adjective check list [Udry and Talbert, 1988]. Another study involving female co-residential students showed that self-reported status position in relation to the peer group was positively correlated with basal TE levels [Cashdan, 1995]. Two of the laboratory experiments mentioned above [van Honk et al., 1999, Josephs et al., 2003] involved female subjects and showed a similar relationship between dominance and endogenous TE levels.

The relationship between TE and prosocial status-seeking behaviours such as leadership behaviour has received little attention so far. Because leadership is associated with the ability to influence others, it seems plausible that TE may be involved in regulating who is more likely to behave more dominantly in such high status positions. There is some evidence supporting this logic in research on adolescent boys [Rowe et al., 2004]. The study found that TE levels were positively correlated with an average of self and parent ratings of leadership, but only among boys in prosocial environments (operationalised as an absence of deviant peers). Among those boys in antisocial environments (operationalised as definitely having deviant peers), TE was unrelated to leadership. This study is important because it suggests that TE may be associated with prosocial behaviours such as leadership, at least for individuals in prosocial environments.

Reciprocal relationship Another important aspect of the theory put forward by Mazur and Booth [1998] is that TE not only affects behaviour but also responds to it. This bidirectional relationship seems to be highly dependent on individual differences in social perception, previous experience as well as the demand of the social context for particular behaviours [Booth et al., 2006]. According to this *reciprocal model*, dominant behaviours or dominance disputes cause TE levels to change, and these changes in TE then feed back to reinforce or discourage further acts of dominance [Mazur and Booth, 1998]. There is ample evidence supporting this model. For example, studies of real-world sports competitions and rigged laboratory competitions have shown that winner's TE levels increase relative to that of losers for a few hours following a competition [Mazur et al., 1992, Mazur and Lamb, 1980, Mccaul et al., 1992], although additional studies suggest that the effect of wins and losses on TE changes depend on personality dispositions [Schultheiss and Stief, 2005]. Studies also provide support for the feed-back aspect of the model - that these temporary changes in TE after competing influence subsequent competitive behaviours [Mehta and Josephs, 2006]. Because of this reciprocal relationship between behaviour and testosterone secretion, it is particularly important to perform

2.3. Neuroendocrine modulation

TE administration studies to investigate the role of TE in social behaviour. Only one study investigated the influence of TE administration on social behaviour in a laboratory setting so far [Pope et al., 2000]. In the task employed [Cherek et al., 1996], a given player A can either increase his own payoff by pressing a button A, or reduce another (fictitious) player B's payoff by pressing a button B. In this study, gradually increasing doses of TE cypionate or placebo were administered over the course of several weeks (150 mg/week for two weeks, 300 mg/week for two weeks and 600 mg/week for two weeks) and decision-making behaviour was tested at the end of the respective substance administration cycle. TE treatment (compared to placebo) resulted in a significantly higher number of button B presses. The experimental design of this study was disadvantageous due to a number of factors. First, TE cypionate was administered over several weeks and might have influenced experiences outside the laboratory. These experiences might have confounded the behavioural measure in the task. Second, the doses of TE that were used led to changed parameters in the hypothalamo-pituitary axis (the authors reported significant suppression of FSH, LH and prolactin concentrations; see also discussion section 5.5.4 on page 98). These confounds prevent us from learning about the causal role of TE effects on behaviour. Third, subjects were deceived (*i.e.* the interacting partner was fictitious). Therefore, in essence, the behavioural measure reported in this study cannot be considered as social decision making according to our operationalisation (see section 1).

The public's view about testosterone The well known fact that males have much higher circulating levels of TE than women likely contributed to the formation of public beliefs about this hormone. It can be assumed that people associate the hormone with the stereotype "manliness", which includes physical attributes such as body strength but also behaviours such aggressiveness, dominance, and impulsivity. In addition, the public's view about TE was certainly also influenced by reports in the news media describing homicides committed by athletes who abused anabolic steroids. Following the publication of a study in the late eighties showing that androgen abuse may lead to psychiatric conditions including manic episodes, major depression and even delusions and hallucinations [Pope and Katz, 1988], the issue received attention on the part of defence lawyers. They described individuals who committed homicide while taking steroids, hoping to improve their legal positions in court. Pope and Katz [1990] described three men who impulsively committed crimes while taking anabolic steroids and who successfully used steroid induced rage (*'roid rage'*) as a legal defence. These issues suggest that the general public has endorsed the view that TE causes aggression, violence, and anti-social behaviour. However, these cases are anecdotes and not scientific evidence. So far, there is one study available showing results that reflect the public's view about TE. Following a double-blind, placebo controlled TE administration, participants had to fill out questionnaires assessing their mood [Bjorkqvist et al., 1994]. A third control group received no substance and subjects in this group were also informed about the fact that they neither received TE nor placebo. The authors found that self-reported anger, irritation, impulsivity and frustration scores were higher in subjects who received *placebo* compared to the TE group or the control group. These results suggest that TE administration may raise expectations, rather than an actual increase in anger and irritability.

2.3.5 Summary

Neuroendocrinology is a relatively old discipline [Carmody, 2008]. Previously, a vast number of behavioural experiments using TE administration have been conducted, mostly in rodents, generally showing an increase in social aggression. Nonetheless, relatively little is known about this hormone's role in human social behaviour. The bulk of studies available on the topic is correlative, whereby TE is measured in saliva or blood, and levels are correlated with (social) behaviour. However, TE can also be injected or applied sublingually, with a cyclodextrin carrier system. The latter is favorable, since it is non-invasive as opposed to injections and does therefore not produce stress in subjects. After sublingual application, blood levels of TE rise quickly and reach its peak after 15 min. The time between maximum serum concentration and appearance of behavioural effects is delayed, perhaps due to the fact that the conventional genomic pathway is slow. Research on this matter in females has established a time-lag of approximately 4 h. Due to its lipophilic nature, non-SHBG bound TE crosses the BBB easily and changes in circulating TE levels reflect changes in TE concentration within the CNS. In humans, increasing TE levels have been associated mainly with dominant or status seeking behaviour. Opposed to this stands the public view that TE causes aggressive, violent, and anti-social behaviour. However, no study has yet investigated the role of TE administration in a social decision making paradigm that involves real interacting partners bargaining over money and no study has assessed the impact of public beliefs about TE on social decision making.

Part II

Empirical Part

Chapter 3

Study 1: Time-course of "off-line" prefrontal rTMS effects – a PET study

3.1 Contributions

Experimental design was done by Daria Knoch and me. Data collection and data analysis was done by me. Daria Knoch coauthored the paper that resulted from this study. The comments about this study were written by me (section 3.7).

3.2 Introduction

TMS has become an indispensable investigation tool in cognitive neuroscience. Its ability to transiently disrupt normal function of human brain regions makes it a unique tool for studying the causal contribution of different brain areas to behaviour. A very promising approach is the application of low frequency rTMS for several min before performing a given task in order to partially elude the unspecific effects of concurrent rTMS stimulation [Abler et al., 2005, Pascual-Leone et al., 1998, Robertson et al., 2003]. This approach, also referred to as "off-line" rTMS, has been used extensively in recent years. It has been applied, *inter alia*, to study parietal contributions to spatial attention [Hilgetag et al., 2001] and spatial hearing [Lewald et al., 2002], or prefrontal contributions to visual working memory [Mottaghy et al., 2002], affective processes [d'Alfonso et al., 2000] and decision making [Knoch et al., 2006b].
Despite considerable advances in this field of research, cognitive neurosciences still

rely primarily on the use of functional imaging. Imaging experiments, however, do not allow drawing firm conclusions about the nature of neural network nodes: activation could be spuriously correlated with task performance and not necessary for proper task execution [Sack and Linden, 2003, Sack et al., 2005, 2007, Walsh and Cowey, 2000]. rTMS seems to be a method well suited for studying the functional relevance of a cortical region, which has been previously identified by a functional imaging experiment, for a specific cognitive function [Hallett, 2007].

When designing an experiment using "off-line" low frequency rTMS, several aspects should be considered. First, the duration of the "off-line" disruptive effect restricts the number of trials in an experiment and, hence, the data collection. Previous studies [d'Alfonso et al., 2000, Mottaghy et al., 2002, Robertson et al., 2001] have provided some information about the duration of behavioural effects after low frequency "off-line" long-train rTMS applied to the DLPFC. The findings of these studies led to the formulation of a rule of thumb: The duration of the after effects is generally half the duration of the stimulation train [Robertson et al., 2003]. However, these studies only report behavioural measures and provide no information about the duration of the neurophysiological effect of "off-line" low frequency rTMS applied to the PFC. Second, stimulation of the homologue contralateral region as a control stimulation site has proven to be an expedient strategy for the control of the side effects of rTMS intervention. Likewise, the side effects of rTMS intervention that ultimately influence the outcome variable are similar. rTMS induces muscle-twitches and tickling sensations at the stimulation site. Especially when rTMS is applied to frontal regions, it causes discomfort, constituting a possible confounding effect [Abler et al., 2005]. As these side effects typically are equally present in the homologue contralateral region one can control for them by also stimulating this region. Thus, if - for example - the stimulation of the right DLPFC causes a behavioural change in task performance while the stimulation of the left DLPFC does not, this effect cannot be attributed to the side effects of rTMS. However, a contralateral control stimulation is only reasonable if a unilateral stimulation leads to unilateral, and not bilateral neurophysiological "off-line" effects. It is therefore important to know whether "off-line" rTMS leads to unilateral or bilateral lasting effects. Third, related to the second point, one should consider that applying rTMS to a given brain region not only affects the target site itself, but also brain areas effectively connected to the target area. Such remote effects evoked by low frequency rTMS over prefrontal areas have been shown in several studies [Kimbrell et al., 2002, Knoch et al., 2006c, Nahas et al., 2001, Ohnishi et al., 2004, Speer et al., 2003]. These studies, however, differed from the usual "off-line" protocol in that ei-

ther rCBF [Nahas et al., 2001, Speer et al., 2003] or glucose uptake [Kimbrell et al., 2002] was measured "online", (*i.e.*, during rTMS application) or in that the duration of the stimulation trains were shorter than usual in the "off-line" approach [Knoch et al., 2006c, Ohnishi et al., 2004].
Despite the wide-spread use of "off-line" rTMS in cognitive tasks, and more recently, social cognitive neuroscience, no experiment has ever investigated the time-course of the neurophysiological lasting effects after a single train of low-frequency rTMS applied to the PFC. We specifically designed our study to assess the issues mentioned above. We were particularly interested in the after effects of right sided prefrontal stimulation as we previously found lateralised behavioural effects using this stimulation protocol [Knoch et al., 2006a]. We used $H_2^{15}O$ PET to assess the effects of rTMS on rCBF. An advantage of this imaging technique is the possibility to compare the relative size of regional blood flow across different brain regions and over time. We applied one single train of low-frequency rTMS to the right DLPFC of twelve subjects and subsequently performed eight sequential $H_2^{15}O$ PET scans.

3.3 Materials and methods

3.3.1 Subjects

Twelve healthy right-handed male subjects [25.3 ± 4.0 years, mean $\pm$ standard deviation (SD)] participated in the study that the local ethics committee approved. All subjects provided written informed consent. Subjects had no history of psychiatric illness or neurological disorder and were naive to TMS.

3.3.2 PET procedures

We used $H_2^{15}O$ PET as a measure of regional synaptic activity. Eight sequential scans were performed in each subject (one baseline scan, seven post stimulation scans). PET scans were acquired on a whole-body scanner (DLS GE Medical Systems, Waukesha, WI) in 3D mode with a 15-cm axial field of view. In each scan, 300 - 400 MBq $H_2^{15}O$ were administered as a bolus using a remotely controlled injection device. Injection of the $H_2^{15}O$ bolus was initiated with an automatic preparation and pump system 30 s before the start of the actual $H_2^{15}O$ PET scan. The accumulated radioactivity counts over 60 s were then taken as measure for cerebral blood flow. Data were reconstructed into 35 image planes with a resolution of 7 mm full width at half maximum (FWHM). Subject preparation included the insertion of an indwelling cubital vein catheter for injection of the $H_2^{15}O$. In order to ensure complete head fixation, the head of the subject was confined in a vacuum cushion. The scan room was darkened and subjects wore foam earplugs for hearing protection. One low-dose CT scan for attenuation correction was performed at the beginning of the experiment, which was immediately followed by the baseline $H_2^{15}O$ scan. Subjects kept their eyes closed during all scans. The remaining seven scans were divided into two blocks. Each block consisted of three and four scans, respectively (Figure 3.1). The order of the two blocks was pseudorandomised across subjects.

3.3.3 Location of the target region

For the exact localisation of the stimulation site, a T1- weighted MRI was acquired for all subjects prior to the PET-experiment. The right DLPFC was located based on fixed coordinates: $x = 39$, $y = 37$, $z = 22$, radius $= 6$ in Talairach space. These coordinates were then transformed to each subject's native brain space using Brainvoyager QX 1.6 software (Brain Innovation BV, Maastricht, NL). The real-time neuronavigation option for Brainvoyager QX 1.6 with the Zebris CMS20S measuring system for real-time motion analysis (Zebris Medical GmbH, Isny, GE) allowed correct placement of the TMS coil in space.

3.3.4 rTMS procedure

rTMS was applied to the right DLPFC for 15 min before each PET scanning block (see Figure 3.1). A Magstim Rapid 2 Stimulator (Magstim, Winchester, USA) and a commercially available figure-of-eight-coil (70 mm diameter double circle, air-cooled) was used. Intensity of stimulation was set to 54% maximum stimulator output. The coil was held tangentially to the subject's head with the handle pointing rostrally. Each subject received one train of 15 min duration at 1 Hz (900 pulses) before each block of PET scanning, amounting to a total of 1800 pulses per session and subject. The time interval between the two stimulation blocks was 30 min. The rTMS parameters employed were well within recommended safety guidelines [Wassermann et al., 1998].

3.3.5 Image analysis

All images were processed using Statistical Parametric Mapping software SPM99 (Wellcome Department of Imaging Neuroscience, UCL, UK. http://www.fil.ion.ucl.uk/spm). Image processing was performed as follows: Head movements were cor-

3.3. Materials and methods

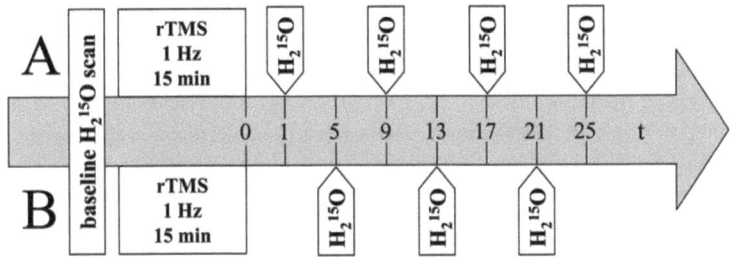

Figure 3.1: Experimental design. To achieve a virtual time resolution of 4 min between $H_2^{15}O$ scans, we set up an interleaved scanning procedure. In every session (A, B), each scanning sequence was preceded by a baseline scan, which was followed by 15 min of 1 Hz rTMS at a fixed intensity of 54% maximum stimulator output and either scanning block A or B. Time points (in min after rTMS train) of $H_2^{15}O$ scans are indicated within the grey arrow. t = time.

rected using the least-squares method and images were then normalised into stereotaxic space [Montreal Neurological Institute coordinates (MNI) as provided by SPM-99] by bilinear interpolation using a PET template. Scans were smoothed using a Gaussian filter of 15 mm in-plane and axial FWHM in order to improve the signal to noise ratio. To remove the effect of global differences in cerebral blood flow between scans, a subject-specific ANCOVA scaling of global activity to a mean of 50 ml/100 g/min was applied.

3.3.6 Region of interest analysis

We performed whole-brain analyses after 1, 5, 9, 13, 17, 21 and 25 min to determine the contrast with the largest rCBF response to low-frequency rTMS. Based on these analyses, the contrast "1 min > baseline" was used to determine regions of interest (ROIs) in the PFC (see Table 3.1; for rCBF increases or decreases in other than prefrontal cortical regions please see Table 3.2 and Table 3.3). Analysis of later time points did not reveal additional clusters of either significantly increased or decreased rCBF. The ROIs were defined as follows: for the stimulation site, a spherical ROI was defined (MNI- coordinates, radius and volume of ROI: x = 50, y = 48, z = 16; radius = 7 mm, volume = 339 mm^3). A second spherical ROI was created in the right VLPFC (x = 42, y = 42, z = -8; radius = 7 mm, volume = 339 mm^3) and a third spherical ROI was created in the right inferior frontal sulcus (x = 32, y

= 36, z = 20; radius = 7 mm, volume = 339 mm^3). Three homotopic contralateral ROIs were defined by mirroring the ROIs in the right hemisphere using MARSBAR [Brett et al., 2002]. In order to control for unspecific arousal effects [Critchley et al., 2000], please see discussion section), two additional control regions were defined in the cerebellum (ipsilaterally: x = 32, y = -70, z = -41 and contralaterally: x = -32, y = -70, z = -41; both 16936 mm3). ROIs were then normalised to baseline and analysed using SPSS version 13.0 (SPSS, Inc., Chicago, IL, USA). A two-way repeated measures analysis of variance (ANOVA) was calculated for each region with the factors: "hemisphere" (left/right) and "time" (1, 5, 9, 13, 17, 21 and 25 min).

3.3.7 Masked correlation analysis

Subject specific time-courses were derived from the right DLPFC and the control region (left/right cerebellum) using MARSBAR [Brett et al., 2002]. These individual time-courses were then incorporated as covariates of interest (correlation analysis). The linear association between rCBF at every time-point and each value derived from the ROI in the right DLPFC and the control region was tested on a voxel-by-voxel basis using the SPM covariates option. To focus only on those regions within the PFC that showed significant rCBF changes in response to "offline" low frequency rTMS, the correlation analysis of rCBF in the right DLPFC was subsequently masked by the subtraction contrast "1 min > baseline" ($P < 0.001$, corresponding to a single-voxel threshold of $t > 3.22$). Threshold in the correlation analysis was set at $P < 0.001$, corresponding to a single-voxel threshold of $t > 3.22$.

3.4 Results

3.4.1 Time-course of "off-line" prefrontal rTMS effects on rCBF

The contrast "1 min > baseline" revealed a significant rCBF increase at the stimulation site ($P < 0.05$, corrected for multiple comparisons over the whole brain). Figure 3.2 illustrates the anatomical coordinates of the stimulation site chosen for navigation and the corresponding region of increased rCBF. The contrasts at other time-points (*i.e.* 5, 9, 13, 17, 21, 25 min after rTMS) showed no significant rCBF effects compared to baseline ($P < 0.05$, corrected for multiple comparisons over the whole brain). After having identified the time-point where rTMS effects were most prominent, we used this contrast to define ROIs for further analysis. Besides the activation cluster at the stimulation site, increased rCBF was present in two other prefrontal areas, *i.e.* in the VLPFC (BA47) and in the inferior frontal sulcus (BA46/48) which were all located ipsilateral to the stimulation site ($P < 0.001$, uncorrected; see Table 3.1). These three regions were then defined as ROIs as described in the methods section.

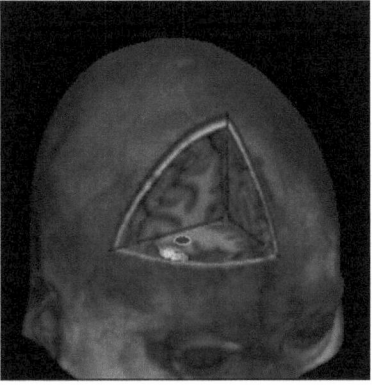

Figure 3.2: Three-dimensional illustration depicts the chosen stimulation coordinates ($x = 39$, $y = 37$, $z = 22$; radius = 6) and the locus of significant increase in rCBF at the stimulation site. Blue spot, stimulation coordinates; orange spot, significantly increased rCBF.

The two-way repeated measures ANOVA revealed a significant main effect of "time" ($F = 2.98$, $df = 6,66$; $P = 0.01$) and "hemisphere" ($F = 6.62$, $df = 1,11$; $P = 0.03$) in the stimulated region. Importantly, the "hemisphere"x"time" interaction was significant ($F = 6.40$, $df = 6,66$; $P < 0.001$), indicating that the stimulated region shows a time effect of rCBF that is specific to one hemisphere [Figure 3.3 (**A**)]. In the VLPFC, a significant main effect of "hemisphere" ($F = 15.09$, $df = 1,11$; $P = 0.003$), but not "time" ($F = 1.44$, $df = 6,66$; $P = 0.21$) was identified. As in the DLPFC, the "hemisphere"x"time" interaction was also significant in the VLPFC ($F = 2.68$, $df = 6,66$; $P = 0.02$) [Figure 3.3 (**B**)]. In the inferior frontal sulcus, a significant main effect of "hemisphere" ($F = 5.72$, $df = 1,11$; $P = 0.04$) was identified. However, neither the main effect of "time" ($F =$

1.38, df = 6,66; P = 0.24) nor the interaction term ("hemisphere"x"time") was significant (F = 0.49, df = 6,66; P = 0.81) [Figure 3.3 (**A**)]. Thus, this region shows a hemispheric rCBF effect that is not time specific [Figure 3.5 (**A**)]. In the control region (cerebellum), the main effect of "hemisphere" was not significant (F = 3.275, df = 1,11; P = 0.098), while the main effect of "time" was significant (F = 3.28, df = 6,66; P = 0.007) [Figure 3.3 (**B**)]. The interaction effect "hemisphere"x"time" was not significant (F = 1.39, df = 6,66; P = 0.23), suggesting that there is no time effect of rCBF specific to one hemisphere in the control region [Figure 3.5 (**B**)]. In summary, these findings suggest a spatially and temporally well described specific "off-line" effect of prefrontal rTMS on blood flow in the DLPFC (BA45/46) and the VLPFC (BA47).

Table 3.1: Prefrontal brain regions that show significantly increased rCBF 1 min after rTMS.

Brain region	BA	Hemisphere	MNI coordinates x y z	T value
DLPFC[†]	BA 45/46	R	44 44 -1	8.31
VLPFC[‡]	BA 47	R	42 42 -8	4.39
Inferior frontal sulcus	BA 46/48	R	32 36 20	3.77

BA, Brodmann area; R, right.

[†] Maxima of regional increases in normalised rCBF based on the contrast "1 min < baseline" (P < 0.05, corrected for multiple comparisons over the whole brain).

[‡] Maxima of regional increases in normalised rCBF based on the contrast "1 min<baseline" (P < 0.001, uncorrected).

Figure 3.4 shows the results of the masked correlation analysis. A significant positive correlation of the time-course of activity in the stimulated region with the time-course of activity in the VLPFC (BA47) was revealed (T = 8.31). We found no regions that showed significant negative correlations in the PFC (Table 3.4). Moreover, we found no significant correlation between the time-course of rCBF in the control region (left/right cerebellum) with the time-course of rCBF in the DLPFC (BA45/46).

In summary, we found increased rCBF in the stimulated area, *i.e.*, DLPFC (BA45/46) and in two other prefrontal regions ipsilateral to the stimulated site: the VLPFC

3.5. Discussion

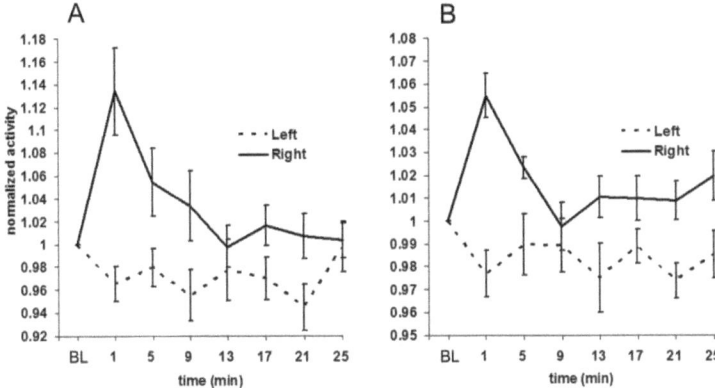

Figure 3.3: The time-course (1 to 25 min) of mean normalised activity (± SEM) in the stimulated area [x = 50, y = 48, z = 16; BA45/46; (**A**)] and in the VLPFC [x = 42, y = 42, z = -8; BA47; (**B**)]. BL, baseline.

(BA47) and the inferior frontal sulcus. These regions showed a strong increase in rCBF immediately after rTMS that returned to baseline within 9 min. Moreover, we found that the time-course of rCBF in the VLPFC(BA47) is correlated with the time-course of rCBF in the stimulated area.

3.5 Discussion

This study examined the neurophysiological effect of one long-duration train of low frequency rTMS applied to the right DLPFC. By sequentially measuring rCBF after prefrontal stimulation we were able to investigate three issues in this study: (1) the duration of the "off-line" neurophysiological effect, (2) whether unilateral prefrontal stimulation leads to unilateral or bilateral "off-line" effects and (3) the effects of low frequency rTMS on remotely connected areas.

The most prominent increase in rCBF was found 1 min after the rTMS train in the right DLPFC (BA45/46) and in the right VLPFC (BA47). While other studies found effects with a delay of several min after cessation of the rTMS train [Chouinard et al., 2003, Johnson et al., 2007], we did not find significantly changed rCBF at later time points, as revealed by whole-brain analyses. One possible explanation is that in the former study a different brain region was stimulated (the left primary

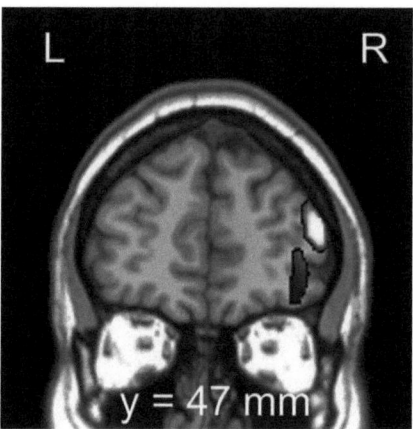

Figure 3.4: The time-course of rCBF in the VLPFC (BA47) correlates positively with the time-course of rCBF in the stimulated area (BA45/46). Results are displayed on a coronal section (y = 47 mm) of averaged anatomical MRI scans (correlation analysis displayed at $P < 0.001$, uncorrected; masked with the contrast "1 min > baseline" at $P < 0.001$, uncorrected). L, left; R, right.

and premotor cortex) while in the latter study behavioural effects and not rCBF were reported after low frequency rTMS of the left DLPFC. In our study, ROI analysis revealed that increased rCBF in the right DLPFC (BA45/46) and right VLPFC (BA47) showed a similar decay over time and returned to baseline values within 9 min. It is possible that the observed rCBF change is the result of unspecific arousal or pain due to rTMS. The cerebellum has previously been reported to positively co-vary with experimentally induced cardiovascular arousal [Critchley et al., 2000]. Additionally, it has been reported to be activated during capsaicine induced pain [May et al., 1998]. To exclude that no such unspecific effects confounded our results, we additionally analysed rCBF in both cerebellar hemispheres and found no "hemisphere"x"time" interaction. Moreover, we found no significant correlation of the time-course of rCBF in the cerebellum as our control region with the time-course of rCBF at the stimulation site (BA45/46). It thus seems that low frequency rTMS indeed induced a temporally well circumscribed "off-line"-rCBF effect on the DLPFC (BA45/46) and the VLPFC (BA47) in our experiment. Thus, as a first conclusion, we find the general rule of thumb confirmed: the effects of 15 min of low frequency rTMS applied to the right DLPFC last approximately half the duration

3.5. Discussion

of the stimulation train. One has to keep in mind, however, that with rCBF we measured indirectly neuronal activity. It might be that rTMS affected neuronal activity for a longer duration and in other regions. Moreover, rCBF was measured while subjects were in a resting state. The effects of "off-line" rTMS on rCBF might be different depending on whether the targeted brain region is involved in the execution of a task or not.

Our results show that stimulating the right DLPFC "off-line" leads to unilateral prefrontal but not bilateral effects on blood flow. Most studies that applied rTMS either "off-line" or "on-line" to the DLPFC found no effect under the site of stimulation [Kimbrell et al., 2002, Ohnishi et al., 2004, Speer et al., 2003]. In one study however, low frequency rTMS was applied to the left DLPFC and a bilateral activation in the DLPFC was found during stimulation [Nahas et al., 2001]. In contrast to this, we measured rCBF "off-line" and found only ipsilateral prefrontal activation clusters. As a second conclusion, we therefore argue that experimental paradigms in cognitive neuroscience which plan to use "off-line" low frequency rTMS to affect the functional integrity of an area in the PFC could employ a contralateral control stimulation to avoid a side-effects bias.

By measuring rCBF sequentially, we were able to show that the time-course of rCBF in the right VLPFC (BA47) is positively correlated with the time-course of rCBF at the stimulation site (BA45/46). Within the PFC, the region in BA47 is the only one that shows a time-course that is correlated with the one in the stimulated area. This finding corroborates the hypothesis of connectivity between dorsal (BA45/46) and ventral aspects (BA47) of the frontal lobes [Petrides and Pandya, 1999]. The VLPFC plays an important role in cognitive neuroscience, such as in decision making [Sakagami and Pan, 2007] or emotion regulation [Ochsner et al., 2004]. A direct stimulation of this brain area involves great discomfort for the volunteer. As a third conclusion, we thus propose that "off-line" long-train low frequency rTMS applied to the right DLPFC can be readily used to target remote connected areas, such as the VLPFC via indirect stimulation.

Interestingly, we only found lasting rCBF increases (and not decreases) in the PFC. At first sight, this seems difficult to reconcile with studies showing a decrease in cortical excitability after long-train low frequency rTMS [Chen et al., 1997, Gerschlager et al., 2001, Kosslyn et al., 1999, Maeda et al., 2000, Muellbacher et al., 2000, Wassermann et al., 1998]. It is important to note, however, that these findings were exclusively based on studies in primary motor or primary visual cortex.

It is assumed that rTMS as employed in our study induces long-term depression (LTD) [Hallett, 2000, Thickbroom, 2007]. Since it has been suggested that rCBF changes reflect (pre)synaptic activity changes [Jueptner and Weiller, 1995], one could expect a decrease in rCBF after LTD induction by low frequency rTMS. While the chosen TMS protocol might indeed have induced a decrease in excitability in the stimulated region, it also might have evoked compensatory regulatory responses in order to maintain normal brain function, which in turn could account for the observed increase.

On the other hand, the observed increased rCBF might also reflect an active inhibition process requiring energy [Ackermann et al., 1984]. This interpretation, however, implies that low frequency rTMS as used in the current study increases the activity of inhibitory interneurons. As several studies suggested, low-frequency rTMS of the primary motor cortex does not lead to increased intracortical inhibition as revealed by subsequent paired-pulse TMS [Brighina et al., 2005, Daskalakis et al., 2006, Fitzgerald et al., 2002, Romero et al., 2002]. Based on this evidence it seems less likely that the observed increased rCBF results from an active inhibition process induced by low-frequency rTMS. Irrespective of the underlying physiological mechanisms, one can assume that rTMS application induces a "virtual lesion" simply by adding neural noise to the system [Husain et al., 2002, Walsh and Cowey, 2000, Walsh and Rushworth, 1999]. The observed increase in rCBF could then again be interpreted as a regulatory response with a time-course reflecting the duration of the "virtual lesion" effect.

3.6 Supplementary material

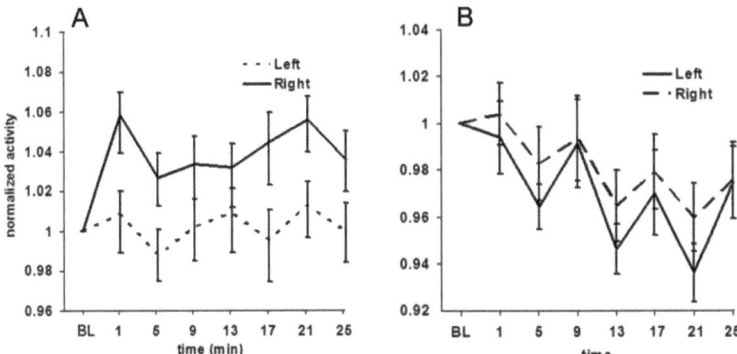

Figure 3.5: The time-course (1 to 25 min) of mean normalised activity (± SEM) in the inferior frontal sulcus [x = 32, y = 36, z = 20; (**A**)] and in the cerebellum [x = 32, y = -70, z = -41; (**B**)]. Please note that the time-course of rCBF in these regions does not correlate with the time-course of rCBF in the stimulated region (BA45/46). BL, baseline.

Table 3.2: Clusters of significant rCBF increase 1 min after stimulation compared to baseline (P < 0.001, uncorrected).

Brain region	Side	T value	MNI coordinates		
			x	y	z
Prefrontal cortex					
DLPFC (BA45/46)	R	5.31	50	48	16
VLPFC (BA47)	R	4.39	42	42	-8
Inferior frontal sulcus (BA46/48)	R	3.77	32	36	20
Other					
Precentral gyrus (BA6/44)	R	5.06	58	8	28
Posterior insula	R	4.84	38	-18	-4
Paracentral lobule	L	4.42	-12	-42	68
Supramarginal gyrus	L	3.76	56	-22	32
Putamen	R	3.71	30	10	-4
Anterior insula	L	3.64	-30	8	8
Operculum	R	3.49	50	14	4
Supplementary motor area	R	3.41	6	-16	56

Table 3.3: Clusters of significant rCBF decrease 1 min after stimulation compared to baseline (P < 0.001, uncorrected).

Brain region	Side	T value	MNI coordinates		
			x	y	z
Parahippocampal gyrus	R	4.40	26	-4	-36
Temporal pole	R	4.09	18	12	-40
Middle temporal gyrus	L	3.92	-66	-54	-12
Lingual gyrus	L	3.71	-26	-60	0
Precuneus	R	3.50	28	-56	0

3.6. Supplementary material

Table 3.4: Brain regions which show a time-course of rCBF that negatively correlates with the time-course of rCBF in the stimulated region. Results are listed based on the correlation analysis ($P < 0.001$, uncorrected), masked with the contrast baseline > 1 min ($P < 0.001$, uncorrected).

Brain region	Side	T value	MNI coordinates*		
			x	y	z
Parahippocampal gyrus	R	4.33	25	-6	-36
Lingual gyrus	R	4.13	-25	-63	4

* coordinates of peak cluster T value in correlation analysis ($P < 0.001$), masked with contrast 1 min $>$ baseline ($P < 0.001$).

3.7 Further comments on Study 1

Summary of main findings There are three main results of the study presented in this chapter. First, 15 min of "off-line" low frequency rTMS of the right DLPFC leads to rCBF changes in the PFC which last approximately half the duration of the stimulation train itself. Second, right dorsolateral prefrontal stimulation leads to ipsilateral prefrontal rCBF effects. Third, low-frequency rTMS of the dorsal aspects of the frontal lobe (BA45/46) leads to rCBF changes in areas assumed to be effectively connected with the stimulation site, such as the VLPFC (BA47).

These findings will be briefly discussed in the context of a recent social decision making experiment that used that same rTMS protocol applied to the same stimulation site as employed in the experiment described in this chapter. Furthermore the often used term "virtual lesion" in the context of *in vivo* experiments will be discussed in the context of a recent *in vitro* study.

3.7.1 "Off-line" rTMS of the DLPFC and social decision making

The first study that reported on the neuroanatomical correlates of responder behaviour in the *Ultimatum Game* [Sanfey et al., 2003] reported that both the anterior insula and the lateral PFC (bilaterally) are more strongly activated when responders face unfair offers compared to when they face fair offers. Since fMRI data are correlative, the causal role of the lateral PFC in influencing responder behaviour is unclear. A recent rTMS experiment aimed to overcome the correlation-causation problematic with respect to the results reported by Sanfey et al. [2003]. They applied "off-line" rTMS to the dorsolateral prefrontal cortices of 52 subjects (left DLPFC, n = 17; right DLPFC, n = 19; sham, n = 16) who were in the role of the responder in an anonymous *Ultimatum Game* with a stake size of CHF 20. They limited the proposer's strategy space, meaning that only offers of CHF 10, 8, 6, or 4 were possible. Obviously CHF 10 is the fair offer, because it splits the stake size equally, while CHF 4 is the most unfair offer. The authors suggest that inhibition of a pre-potent response may be relevant for the responder behaviour in the *Ultimatum Game* because he/she faces two competing goals: a fairness goal (to punish the proposer for having made unfair offers) and self-interest (to keep the money). The question is which motivational impulse should be restrained.

The lateral PFC is generally thought to be involved in executive control, goal maintenance, and the inhibition of pre-potent responses [Miller and Cohen, 2001]. Thus by applying "off-line" low-frequency rTMS to the DLPFC, Knoch et al. [2006b] in-

3.7. Comments on Study 1   51

vestigated whether the transient "virtual lesion" of the lateral PFC will lead to a change in acceptance rate. The results showed that the group receiving rTMS to the right DLPFC has a significantly higher acceptance rate than those receiving rTMS applied to the left DLPFC and those receiving sham rTMS. Because subjects self-reported fairness judgments with regard to different offers were not changed, the authors suggested that subjects who received right prefrontal rTMS are less able to resist the economic temptation to accept even unfair offers.

Since the stimulation coordinates in the experiment presented in this chapter were the same, we may cautiously interpret the data reported by Knoch et al. [2006b] in the light of our findings. Compared to baseline, we found increased rCBF in BA46/48 and BA47 and rCBF was correlated in these two regions over time indicating a possible connectivity. These results fit nicely with those of Knoch et al. [2006b], because although they applied rTMS to the DLPFC, it is rather BA47 (VLPFC, mostly right lateralised) that has been related to inhibitory control functions [Aron et al., 2003]. Therefore, it might be possible that the observed increase in proposer offers were due, in part, by the indirect (transsynaptic) stimulation of the VLPFC via the DLPFC. These two brain regions have been shown to be effectively connected using antero- and retrograde tracers in monkeys [Petrides and Pandya, 1999].

Because we still know little about the neurophysiological processes that underlie *in vivo* and *in vitro* effects of rTMS, an important open question is how the unspecific stimulation of millions of neurons in the target area may result in prolonged "disruption of normal function".

3.7.2 Virtual lesion

A number of papers including the one presented in this chapter use the term "virtual lesion" to refer to the effects of low frequency rTMS applied to the cortex [Sack et al., 2007, George et al., 2002, Knoch and Fehr, 2007]. When TMS is used in single pulse mode, the term might be adequate, since it occurs first because the stimulus transiently synchronises the activity of a large proportion of neurons under the coil and second because it induces a long lasting generalised inhibitory post-synaptic potential that reduces cortical activity for the next $50 - 200$ ms depending on stimulus intensity [Siebner and Rothwell, 2003].

When low frequency rTMS is applied to a cortical area, it might be rather incorrect to speak of a transient "virtual lesion". First, rTMS of a given brain region does not lead to a loss of function. Second, it was proposed that LTD might be the mechanism by which low frequency rTMS induces transient decreases in general excitability of the neuronal networks in the targeted brain area [Sven Bestmann, *personal communication*, Robertson et al., 2003, Hallett, 2000, Thickbroom, 2007]. The observations of decreased cortical excitability after low frequency rTMS are, however, exclusively based on research in the motor system and therefore difficult to apply to prefrontal regions. Furthermore, it is likely that LTD after low frequency rTMS will only occur in a minority of neurons.

The hypothesis that rTMS might cause excitation and LTD by only affecting a minority of the whole population of neurons was recently corroborated by a *in vitro* experiment using single pulse magnetic stimulation (MS) of neuronal cell cultures [Rotem and Moses, 2008]. Using a concentric ring of one-cell layer rat hippocampal neurons, Rotem and Moses [2008] investigated the neuronal network responses to single pulse MS and made two important suggestions based on their findings: first, it is not the total projected length that counts in MS but rather the length of the longest contiguous stretch along the direction of the electric field. For example, a long, but zigzag shaped axon may not be excited by MS. Second, some neurons do not respond at all to MS, even when magnetic field density is doubled. Other neurons respond already at lower intensities. The authors suggested that a subpopulation of initiating neurons contribute to the excitation of the network after MS and that this might indicate that MS is a single neuron phenomenon.

It is important that future *in vitro* studies will also investigate the effects of low frequency MS on neuronal responses. If a possible LTD induction is also restricted to a few initiating neurons one might hypothesise that also a few neurons determine the disruptive effects of low frequency rTMS *in vivo*. Therefore, it might be more correct to speak of a "disruption of normal function" of a brain area rather than of a "virtual lesion".

Chapter 4

Study 2: DRD4 polymorphism predicts the effect of L-DOPA on gambling behaviour

4.1 Contributions

Experimental design, pilot study, data collection were performed by Daria Knoch and me. Data analysis was done by me. Daria Knoch coauthored the paper that resulted from this study. The comments on this study were written by me (section 4.6).

4.2 Introduction

Several lines of evidence link the DAergic system to impulse control [Cools, 2008], and substance addiction [Dalley et al., 2007], as well as to non-substance addictions such as pathological gambling [Bergh et al., 1997]. Anecdotal evidence for the latter comes from numerous case reports describing the development of pathological gambling in Parkinson's disease after initiation of DAergic drug treatment [Voon et al., 2007a]. However, not all individuals with Parkinson's disease are at risk of developing pathological gambling during DAergic treatment. The fact that only a subgroup of Parkinson's disease patients treated with DAergic drugs develops pathological gambling suggests an underlying vulnerability, possibly mediated by genetic factors. Support for this notion derives from research in healthy subjects suggesting that genetic vulnerability for pathological gambling may be linked to variation in the D4 receptor gene [Perez de Castro et al., 1997]. The D4 receptor gene contains a highly polymorphic region within its third exon, also referred to as the DRD4 exon III variable tandem number repeat polymorphism (DRD4 polymorphism) [van Tol et al., 1992]. The polymorphism is an imperfect repeat translated into 16 amino acids found to be present two to eleven times in different alleles of DRD4 [Lichter et al., 1993, Ding et al., 2002]. Presence of the 7R allele has been associated with pathological gambling and other impulse control disorders such as attention-deficit hyperactivity disorder (ADHD) [Faraone et al., 2001, Li et al., 2006]. Furthermore, among individuals with ADHD, the 7R allele has been associated with poor performance on laboratory measures of impulse control as well [Langley et al., 2004]. Poor impulse control and ADHD are both related to pathological gambling [Steel and Blaszczynski, 1998, Specker et al., 1995].

These lines of evidence suggest that both DAergic drug challenge and the DRD4 polymorphism might also influence gambling behaviour measured in the laboratory. In particular, an individuals' behavioural response to a drug challenge might be determined by genetic variation in the DRD4 gene. Up to now, no study has investigated how the interaction of genetic factors with the administration of a DAergic drug affects gambling behaviour. This can only be investigated by using a pharmacogenetic approach.

Building on the evidence mentioned above, we hypothesised that the administration of a DAergic drug has a differential effect on gambling behaviour depending on variation in the D4 receptor gene. In order to explore a gene-drug interaction on gambling behaviour systematically, we used healthy subjects to avoid the confounding effects of Parkinson's disease. We used L-DOPA versus placebo administration to investigate how the presence or absence of the 7R allele determines the impact of DAergic stimulation on gambling behaviour.

4.3 Results

We administered 300 mg of the DA precursor L-DOPA in a double-blind, parallel-groups, placebo-controlled experiment to 205 healthy males. Subjects played 40 trials of a gambling task that was administered 60 min after L-DOPA intake, when the plasma level of L-DOPA reached its peak (mean $\pm$ SEM: 4.35 ± 0.38 mg/l blood serum). These pharmacokinetic parameters were determined in a separate study involving ten healthy young male subjects (Figure 4.2). In the gambling task (see section 4.5), participants opened 6.05 out of ten boxes on average (SD ± 0.82). ANOVA revealed no increase in gambling behaviour associated with L-DOPA compared to placebo administration [$F = 0.81$, $P = 0.37$, see Figure 4.1 (**A**)]. L-DOPA

4.3. Results

administration differed, however, with respect to its impact on gambling behaviour as a function of the subjects' DRD4 polymorphism. We found a significant positive interaction between drug treatment and genotype on gambling behaviour [$F = 5.43$, $P < 0.05$, see Figure 4.1 (**B**)]. Specifically, increased gambling was observed in subjects who carry the 4/7 genotype and who received L-DOPA, but not in those who received L-DOPA and who carry the 4/4 genotype ($t = 3.27$, $P < 0.01$; Cohen's d = 0.90). In contrast, no genotype effect on gambling behaviour was observed in the placebo group ($t = 0.11$, $P = 0.92$).

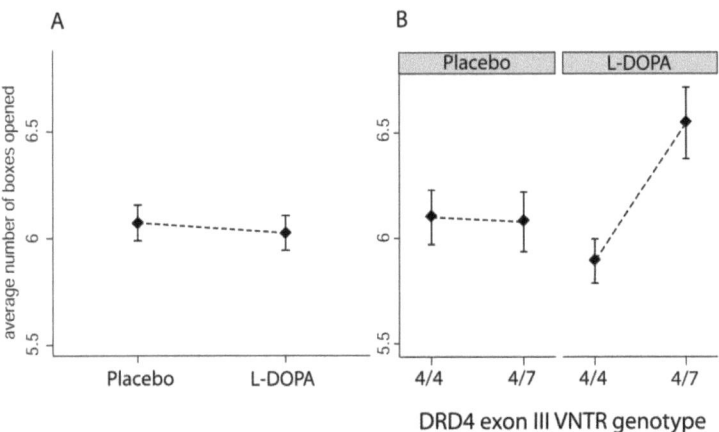

Figure 4.1: Gambling behaviour as indexed on the y axes by the average number of opened boxes over all trials that were ended by the subject voluntarily. (**A**) No increase in gambling behaviour was observed following L-DOPA compared to placebo administration. (**B**) Increased gambling behaviour was observed in subjects who carry the 4/7 genotype of the DRD4 polymorphism and who received L-DOPA but not in those who carry the 4/4 genotype. This genotype effect on gambling behaviour was absent in the placebo group. Error bars indicate SEM.

The observed effect on gambling behaviour was not attributable to side-effects of drug administration. There were no significant drug treatment group differences on measures of side-effects at baseline and before the gambling task was performed (all $P < 0.10$), except for the factor "alertness", for which a marginally significant difference was revealed ($t = 1.68$, $P = 0.09$). However, the interaction term between drug treatment and genotype on gambling behaviour remains significant if

we control for this factor (F = 4.66, P = 0.03).
Because the observed differential drug effect on gambling behaviour could be attributed to pre-existing trait differences in subjects' propensity to act impulsively, we measured subjects' self-reported impulsivity and self-control capacity, at the beginning of the experimental session. However, we found no differences across drug treatment groups for either impulsivity (F = 0.35, P = 0.56), or self-control (F = 1.38, P = 0.24). In addition, the interaction term between drug treatment and genotype on gambling behaviour remains significant if we control for impulsivity and self-control (F = 4.53, P = 0.03). Finally, measures of impulsivity and self-control did not correlate with gambling behaviour (r = -0.01, P = 0.79; r = -0.03, P = 0.64, respectively).

4.4 Discussion

This study is the first to show that individual genetic predispositions predict gambling behaviour in a non-clinical sample in response to the administration of a DAergic drug. Specifically, we found that L-DOPA administration was associated with increased gambling behaviour in carriers of the 4/7 genotype of the DRD4 polymorphism, but not in carriers of the 4/4 genotype. These findings highlight the importance of including genetic information in pharmacological intervention studies investigating behaviour, and might explain the failure of previous attempts to find an effect of DAergic stimulation on gambling behaviour.
Previous association studies have linked the 7R allele of the DRD4 polymorphism with higher self-reported novelty-seeking [Kluger et al., 2002] and laboratory measures of impulsivity [Congdon et al., 2008] in the healthy population. These findings suggest an important role of the D4 receptor in the modulation of inhibitory control processes. Poor inhibitory control has been discussed as a critical vulnerability marker for drug abuse in humans [Verdejo-Garcia et al., 2008] and predicted high doses of cocaine self-administration in rats [Dalley et al., 2007].
Our findings suggest that the relative ability for impulse control as determined by the DRD4 polymorphism genotype might be predictive of whether an individual is able to avoid excessive drug intake after exposure to a DAergic drug. Finally, our results are of clinical relevance for Parkinson's disease patients as the individual DRD4 polymorphism genotype might assist in predicting the probability of developing an impulse control disorder, such as a pathological gambling.

4.5 Methods

4.5.1 Subjects

205 healthy young males with mean ($\pm$ SD) age of 23.5 years ($\pm$ 3.6) took part in a double-blind, placebo controlled experiment that the local ethics committee had previously approved. Standardised interviews, under supervision of a neurologist (P.S.), revealed that the subjects had no significant general psychiatric, medical, or neurological disorders. They were included in the study after having provided written informed consent. Three subjects reported nausea and their data were discarded. Two subjects were excluded from further analysis because they did not understand the instructions.

4.5.2 Experimental procedure

All experiments took place at the experimental laboratory of the Institute for Empirical Research in Economics in Zurich, Switzerland, where a total of ten sessions were conducted. All sessions started at 08:30 a.m. Subjects were randomly assigned to receive either a single dose of 300 mg of Madopar (consisting of 300 mg L-DOPA and 75 mg benserazide, a peripheral DOPA-decarboxylase inhibitor) or a placebo. They then received a standardised meal and 100 ml of water. 12 h (*i.e.* on the evening before the behavioural experiment) and 30 min before L-DOPA administration, subjects were required to ingest 10 mg of domperidone in order to avoid possible peripheral DAergic side effects such as nausea and orthostatic hypotension. After subjects read the instructions, we checked whether they understood the rules of the gambling task by having them answer control questions. With the exception of two subjects, all answered these control questions correctly. To assess potential side effects of L-DOPA treatment, subjects were asked to rate their subjective feelings, using visual analogue scales (VAS). Subjects performed the gambling task 60 min after L-DOPA intake, when the plasma level of L-DOPA reached its peak (Figure 4.2). The task was implemented in zTree software and presented on computer screens [Fischbacher, 2007]. After the gambling task, subjects also filled out personality questionnaires that assessed motor impulsivity [Patton et al., 1995] and self-control [Tangney et al., 2004], and were asked to perform a mouthwash to collect buccal epithelial cells for the preparation of DNA. Subjects received a flat fee of CHF 100 (CHF 1.00 $\approx$ \$ 0.90) for participation in the experiment. Each point in the gambling task was worth CHF 0.25. Payment according to the earned points was done for each subject in private at the end of the experiment.

Chapter 4. Study 2: L-DOPA and gambling behaviour

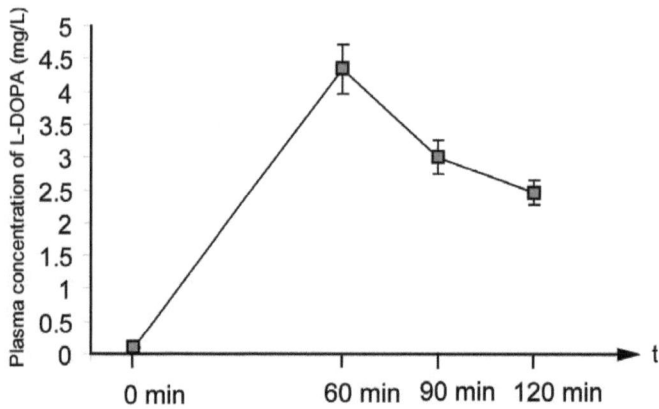

Time after Madopar (300 mg) administration

Figure 4.2: Pharmacokinetics of L-DOPA concentration [mg/l] in serum after oral administration of 300 mg of Madopar to ten healthy young men. Error bars indicate SEM.

4.5.3 Genotyping

Subjects rinsed their mouth with 25 ml of Candida-mouthwash and spit it into sterile 50-ml polypropylene tubes. The samples were stored at 4 °C if they were not to be processed within 2 h of collection. From these samples, DNA was extracted and amplified (Genetica, Zurich, Switzerland).
The following procedure was performed: the tubes were centrifuged at 1600 RCF/g using a Hettich Rotina 46 S centrifuge. The remaining pellet was resuspended in 180 μl ATL and Proteinase K was added (30 μl of a 20-mg/ml stock solution). This solution was hybridised for 3 h at 58°C. Then, the solution was stirred and transferred into a 2 ml test tube. The tube was centrifuged for 1 min at 10'000 rpm. From this a standard EZ1 DNA extraction was performed using the BioRobot EZ1 following the QIAamp Blood Kit Protocol (obtained from Quiagen AG, Hombrechtikon, Switzerland). The obtained DNA concentration was then measured using a photometer (NANODROP, Fisher Scientific GmbH, Schwerte, GE). The exon III repeat region of the DRD4 receptor was characterised by PCR amplification employing the following primers:
F5'-TTCCTACCCTGCCCGCTCATGCTGCTGCTCATCTGG-3'

4.5. Methods

R5'-ACCACCACCGGCAGGACCCTCATGGCCTTGCGCTC-3'

PCR reactions were performed using 5 μl Master Mix (Thermo scientific), 2μl primers (0.5 M), 0.6μl Mg/Cl2 (2.5 mM), 0.4l DMSO 5% and 1l of water to total of 9l total volume and an additional 1l of genomic DNA was added to the mixture. All PCR reactions were employed on a Biometra T1 Thermocycler (Biometra, Goettingen, Germany). PCR reaction conditions were as follows: preheating step at 94.0°C for 5 min, 34 cycles of denaturation at 94.0°C for 30 s, reannealing at 55°C for 30 s and extension at 72°C for 90 s. The reaction proceeded to a hold at 72°C for 5 min. The reaction mixture was then electrophoresed on a 3% agarose gel (AMRESCO) with ethidium bromide to screen for genotypes.

4.5.4 Subject grouping according to the DRD4 exon III VNTR polymorphism genotype

Subjects were grouped according to the two most frequent genotypes (Table 4.1). The 4/4 and the 4/7 genotypes account for the majority of the observed genotypes (64% and 20%, respectively) at a global level [Lichter et al., 1993] and in our sample (47.50% and 21.00%, respectively). We thus compared a group of subjects who are homozygous for the 4R allele (4/4 homozygotes, n = 95) with a group of subjects that carry a 4R and a 7R allele (4/7 heterozygotes, n = 42). As an alternative approach, we grouped subjects according to presence or absence of the 7R allele. In this analysis, we compared a group of subjects who carry at least one 7R allele (n = 54) with those who do not carry the 7R allele (n = 146). This grouping yielded similar results. ANOVA revealed again a significant positive interaction between drug treatment and genotype on gambling behaviour (F = 4.73, P < 0.05). In the L-DOPA group, 7R allele carriers opened significantly more boxes than those who do not carry the 7R allele (t-test, two-sided, t = 2.67, P < 0.01; Cohen's d = 0.63). Again, there was no genotype effect present in the placebo group (t-test, two-sided, t = 0.42, P = 0.68).

Table 4.1: Genotype frequencies for the DRD4 polymorphism, sorted according to frequency.

Genotype	Number of subjects	Frequency
4/4	95	47.5%
4/7	42	21.0%
2/4	32	16.0%
3/4	13	6.5%
2/7	5	2.5%
7/7	5	2.5%
2/2	2	1.0%
3/7	2	1.0%
4/5	2	1.0%
2/5	1	0.5%
3/3	1	0.5%
Total	200	100%

4.5.5 Gambling task

Gambling behaviour was measured by letting subjects play 40 trials of a task, in which the risk associated with acting increases dynamically with each additional action taken [Slovic, 1966]. Figure 4.3 depicts one exemplary trial of the gambling task. In this task, the expected marginal value of opening an additional box (provided one has already successfully opened $n - 1$ boxes) is positive for opening up to five boxes and is negative for opening six boxes or more (see Figure 4.4).

4.5.6 Measures of drug related side effects

VAS were recorded prior to substance administration and just immediately before the gambling task was performed. Items in the scale were alert - drowsy, calm - excited, strong - feeble, muzzy - clear-headed, well coordinated - clumsy, lethargic - energetic, contented - discontented, troubled - tranquil, mentally slow - quick-witted, tense - relaxed, attentive - dreamy, incompetent - proficient, happy - sad, antagonistic - amicable, interested - bored and withdrawn - gregarious. These dimensions were presented as 10 cm lines on a computer screen and volunteers marked their

4.5. Methods

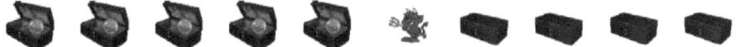

Figure 4.3: One exemplary trial of the gambling task. In each of the 40 trials, subjects were presented with an array of ten closed boxes on a computer screen. In a sequence from left to right, subjects had the possibility of opening box after box (by pressing a button one). They were told that nine boxes contained monetary rewards ("win boxes"), while one box ("loss box") contained a "devil" that would make them lose all the money they had collected in the current trial, simultaneously ending the current trial. Opening a "win box" was associated with a payoff of one point (= 0.25 CHF). After opening a "win box", subjects had to decide whether they wanted to open another box or to terminate the trial (by pressing a button two) and earn all win points. Once the "loss box" was opened, subjects earned nothing for that trial. The "devil" was randomly assigned to one of the ten boxes in each trial, thus, no learning was involved in this task. The average number of boxes opened in those trials that subjects voluntarily terminated served as an indicator of a subject's level of gambling behaviour. In the above example, the subject had won nothing for that trial, since the loss box was opened after successfully opening of five win boxes.

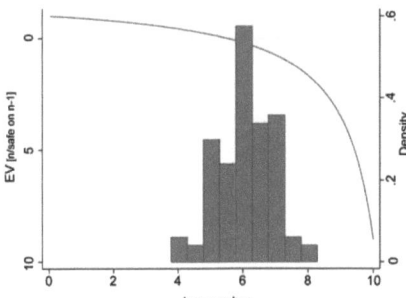

Figure 4.4: The red line depicts the expected marginal value of opening a further box given one has already opened n safe boxes (y axis on the left: EV $[n/safe$ on $n-1]$). Thus, opening more than five boxes is associated with a negative expected marginal value and is considered a risk seeking strategy while opening less than five boxes is considered a risk averse strategy. The histogram (y axis on the right: density) indicates the distribution of the average number of boxes that have been opened by subjects in the *placebo group* in trials where they decided to stop and earn the accumulated points.

current state on each line with a mouse click. In line with previous studies, the factors "alertness", "contentedness", and "calmness" were calculated from these items [Norris, 1971, Chamberlain et al., 2006].

4.5.7 Statistical analysis

The statistical analysis is based on univariate one-way ANOVA. All tests are two-sided tests. We examined the impact of drug [with a binary indicator for drug indicating whether the subject received L-DOPA ($= 1$) or placebo ($= 0$)], the impact of genotype [with a binary indicator for genotype in subjects who carry the 4/7 genotype ($= 1$) and the 4/4 genotype ($= 0$)], and the impact of the interactions between these two variables in an univariate one-way ANOVA on gambling behaviour. In a more detailed analysis, we also incorporated the two trait variables impulsivity and self control.

4.6 Further comments on Study 2

Summary of main findings Using a simple and intuitively comprehensible gambling task, we found that subjects who receive L-DOPA and carry at least one copy of the 7R allele of the DRD4 polymorphism show increased gambling behaviour compared to non-7R carriers. L-DOPA administration was not associated with a change in gambling propensity compared to placebo administration when the DRD4 polymorphism was not considered. Moreover, the DRD4 polymorphism did not predict gambling behaviour in the placebo group. Finally, we did not observe a correlation between self-reported impulsivity and self-control with gambling behaviour. The following discussion begins with a critical evaluation of the gambling task from a sensorimotor perspective. Subsequently, different sections speculate about the potential influence of two brain regions in which both the DRD4 has been reported to be expressed and which are also often reported to be activated during risky decision making: the PFC and the vStr. Since the relative impact of different brain structures cannot be clearly addressed in pharmacogenetic studies investigating behaviour, additional neuroimaging studies may serve this purpose. This combination has, however, inherent pitfalls, which will be discussed. Finally, the findings reported in this chapter will be discussed from a clinical perspective and ethical issues of using pharmacogenetics for individualised treatment in psychiatry will be addressed.

4.6.1 Motor repetitive behaviour

Rylander [1972] first used the term "punding" to describe a distinctive stereotyped behaviour in amphetamine and cocaine addicts. Punding is a peculiar behaviour characterised by an intense fascination with repetitive, purposeless, excessive activities such as the manipulation of technical equipment, handling, examining or sorting through common objects, grooming and hoarding [Friedman, 1994]. These behaviours seem to be similar to the stereotyped behaviours that occur in animals given amphetamine [Ridley and Baker, 1982]. The phenomenon has only recently come to the attention of physicians, since accumulating evidence shows punding in Parkinson's disease patients, triggered by DAergic replacement therapy [Friedman, 1994, Black and Friedman, 2006]. These lines of evidence suggest that punding is related to DAergic stimulation.

The gambling task [Slovic, 1966] presented in this chapter requires two basic motor actions: to press a button one on a computer keyboard to open boxes containing monetary rewards and to press another button two to stop opening boxes and collect the accrued money in the trial. Since subjects opened 6.05 boxes on average (SD = 0.82), they performed seven motor actions on average: six identical actions (button one presses) and one different action (a button two press) at the end of a trial. Thus, if the administration of L-DOPA caused motor repetitive behaviour reminiscent of punding this could have resulted in a more frequent repetition of button one presses compared to placebo administration, appearing as increased gambling propensity. We did, however, not observe a significant difference in gambling behaviour between the two drug treatment groups suggesting that L-DOPA treatment alone did not cause motor repetitive behaviour in the context of the gambling task. If repetitive behaviour were the underlying mechanism by which the 7R carriers contribute to the pharmacogenetic effect on gambling, it would remain to be explained how the different D4 receptor isoforms (the 7R and 4R variants) differentially affect motor repetitive behaviour.

A recent knock-out study in mice suggested that the D4 receptor might play a modulatory role in DAergic drug stimulated motor behaviours. When the D4 receptor was disabled, DA synthesis and the concentration of DA's major metabolite DOPAC (see section 2.2.1) increased in the dorsal striatum and the mice showed locomotor supersensitivity to ethanol, cocaine, and methamphetamine [Rubinstein et al., 1997]. It is a feasible hypothesis that DAergic stimulation also caused increased repetitive behaviours in these D4 receptor knock-out mice, although the authors did not report on stereotypical behaviour specifically. The authors discussed the observed motor hyper-responsiveness to DAergic drugs in the context of the often reported blunted response of the 7R receptor variant to DA (see section 2.2.1). Although speculative, it might therefore also be possible that subjects who carry a 7R allele react with motor repetitive behaviour in response to DAergic stimulation.

4.6.2 DRD4 modulation

Prefrontal cortex and impulse control

Based on the suggestion that the lateral PFC plays an important role in impulse control [Miller and Cohen, 2001, Aron et al., 2003] and the observation that lesions to this structure may cause an increased gambling propensity in the laboratory [Clark et al., 2003, Manes et al., 2002, Floden et al., 2008] suggests an important role of this brain region in influencing gambling behaviour in healthy subjects as well. Moreover, the observation that the absence of DA in PFC is detrimental for its normal function [Brozoski et al., 1979] together with the observation that lateral PFC function may stand in an inverted U-shaped relationship with DA content

4.6. Comments on Study 2

[Vijayraghavan et al., 2007, Cools, 2008] suggests that DAergic modulation of lateral prefrontal cortical function might influence gambling behaviour by causing a deficit in impulse control. In the following, the potential role of poor impulse control as a cause of the observed increase in gambling behaviour will be discussed in the context of the potential role the DRD4 might play herein.

Descriptive model The "overdose" model is a rather descriptive attempt to explain findings of reversal learning deficits in the "on-state" in medicated early Parkinson's disease patients [Gotham et al., 1988, Swainson et al., 2000, Cools et al., 2003]. It states that L-DOPA medication leads to a relative DAergic "overdose" of the vStr, which is projecting to the ventrolateral aspects of the PFC, resulting in diminished impulse control [Cools et al., 2003]. We found, however, no main effect of L-DOPA on gambling behaviour suggesting that the hypothesised DAergic "overdose" of the lateral PFC [Cools et al., 2003] was perhaps not pronounced enough to cause impulse control deficits. It might, however, be possible that only those subjects who have a genetic predisposition for poor impulse control and pathological gambling (the 7R carriers) responded to L-DOPA administration with an increased gambling propensity. In other words, while the DAergic "overdose" of the ventral frontostriatal circuitry might have been insufficient to cause impulse control deficits in non-7R carriers, it might have been sufficient in the 7R carriers. This explanation does, however, not explain how an increased DA concentration might interact with the DRD4 on a mechanistic level.

Mechanistic model A first question that arises is whether the L-DOPA mediated increase in DA levels directly affect the DRD4 in the PFC or whether they are stimulated via the DAergic projections from the striatum to the PFC. To answer this question, we have to know where DA synthesis and storage in the human brain after L-DOPA administration is highest (see section 2.2.1). An early study investigated the distribution of AADC in *post mortem* human brains and reported highest AADC concentration in striatum, the hypothalamus and the ventral tegmental area along with relatively low concentrations in the PFC [Lloyd and Hornykiewicz, 1972]. More recent studies have used either ^{18}F-labelled L-DOPA or ^{11}C-labelled L-DOPA as PET tracers to assess the rate of DA synthesis and storage in the living human brain [Gjedde et al., 1991, Moore et al., 2003, Ito et al., 2008]. These studies generally report a high rate of DA synthesis in the nigrostriatal and mesolimbic DAergic system and a relatively low synthesis in the PFC. In summary, these studies suggest that L-DOPA administration mainly increases DA concentrations in the striatum and less so in the PFC. Therefore, stimulation of the DRD4 in PFC are likely a result from an increased DA concentration in the striatum via its projections to the PFC.

The next question is how a presynaptic DA release impacts on the two DRD4 variants (4R and 7R) and how these are different in modulating PFC function. Although highly speculative, the literature reviewed in section 2.2.1 on page 13 allows the following reasoning. There is evidence that the DRD4 is located in human PFC [Lahti et al., 1997, Primus et al., 1997]. Moreover, there is evidence that the DRD4 is expressed on GABAergic interneurons in primate PFC [Mrzljak et al., 1996] and that DRD4 activation inhibits GABAergic transmission [Wang et al., 2002]. Therefore, less DRD4 activation leads to increased GABAergic transmission in PFC. Molecular biological approaches have shown both an increased and decreased functional potency of the 7R variant compared to the 4R variant [Asghari et al., 1995, van Craenenbroeck et al., 2005, Wedemeyer et al., 2007, Schoots and Van Tol, 2003]. If the 7R variant is less efficient in signal transmission compared to the 4R variant, carriers of the 7R allele would show decreased inhibition of GABAergic signalling and thus increased PFC function. Increasing DAergic transmission and the resulting increase in DRD4 activation should therefore result in a relative improvement of PFC function compared to non-7R carriers. Improved PFC function might result in better impulse control and should, therefore, result in decreased gambling propensity. However, if the 7R variant is more efficient in signal transmission as suggested by Wedemeyer et al. [2007], this were more consistent with the results presented in this chapter.

Given the many uncertainties with respect to the anatomical distribution and functions of the DRD4 in humans, these arguments are purely speculative and the question whether DAergic stimulation of the DRD4 leads to a general improvement or reduction in PFC function remains elusive. Nevertheless, the finding that the DRD4 is located on GABAergic interneurons in PFC suggests its potentially powerful role in modulating PFC function.

Striatum and reward sensitivity

It is generally assumed that DAergic neurons projecting from the vStr to the PFC play a critical role in the anticipation of rewards [Schultz et al., 1997]. As opposed to the many studies that have shown a predominant prefrontal localisation of the DRD4, others have suggested that it is located in the vStr [Svingos et al., 2000, Rivera et al., 2002]. This suggests that the receptor may mediate a direct effect on reward processing. The DRD4, which belongs to the D2-type receptors, exerts an in-

hibitory effect on adenylyl cyclase to and formation of cAMP upon DA binding [Chio et al., 1994, see also section 2.2.1 on page 12]. Because some have suggested that the 7R variant is less efficient in inhibiting cAMP formation [Asghari et al., 1995], the 7R allele carriers may have chronically elevated cAMP levels which might result in a relatively higher baseline activity (or excitability) of the vStr [Hutchison et al., 2002].
A recent imaging genetics study revealed that the presence of the 7R allele was associated with relatively greater vStr reactivity in response to positive and negative feedback-associated monetary rewards [Forbes et al., 2009]. Furthermore, the study has shown that the presence of the 9R allele of the 40 base-pair VNTR DAT polymorphism, which is linked with reduced DAT expression and presumably greater striatal synaptic DA content [Heinz et al., 2000], showed increased vStr activation in the anticipation of the monetary rewards as well. The authors suggested that increased vStr activity might be associated with a relatively increased sensitivity for immediate rewards together with a decreased sensitivity for adverse outcomes [Forbes et al., 2009]. Thus, L-DOPA administration, which increases DA concentration mainly in the striatum [Ito et al., 2008], could have led to a relatively greater increase in vStr activity in 7R allele carriers compared to the 4R carriers. These subjects perhaps placed more weight on the monetary rewards versus potential losses in the gambling task, resulting in the observed increase in gambling propensity.

4.6.3 Self-reported impulsivity and gambling behaviour

The finding that gambling behaviour was not related to self-reported measures of impulsivity and self-control is consistent with previous studies that also failed to observe relations between self-reports and behavioural measures [Crean et al., 2000, Mitchell, 1999]. The lack of such a correlation might be due to the fact that self-report questionnaire based methodology have inherent limitations. Specifically, self-report methods may not reflect the most reliable and accurate data regarding a particular construct, given a number of factors. First, participants may perceive negative consequences as a result of reporting particular behaviours and may therefore not answer truthfully. There also is the possibility that participants lack insight into their behaviour, which could interfere with their ability to provide an accurate report. Finally, individuals might be prone to certain self-perception biases that diverge dramatically from their actual behaviour. Performance on a behavioural task is less sensitive to biased self-perceptions, lack of insight into own behaviour and is less influenced by social desirability.

4.6.4 Specificity of L-DOPA effects

Because Parkinson's disease is associated with a loss of DAergic neurons and L-DOPA supplementation is an efficient strategy to treat the disease, one might expect that L-DOPA administration leads mainly to an increase in DA concentration in the CNS. However, many studies suggest that the effects of L-DOPA administration are by no means uniquely DAergic.

Norepinephrine A study conducted in the seventies suggested that the administration of L-DOPA systemically to rats appears to modify brain NE metabolism. There seems to be a transient increase in brain NE concentration, because some of the L-DOPA that enters the brain is converted to NE and there is an apparent brief acceleration in the turnover of brain NE. These changes occurred when L-DOPA could still be detected in the brain [Chalmers et al., 1971]. However, others have also reported that a very large intraperitoneal dose of L-DOPA (450 mg/kg) did not affect brain NE content [Everett and Borcherding, 1970].

Serotonin Since L-DOPA may act as an inhibitor of TrpH [Naoi et al., 1994], it may interfere with the biochemical conversion of tryptophan to 5-HTP, which is the rate limiting step in 5-HT synthesis. Therefore L-DOPA administration may have a substantial impact on the serotonergic system and it was reported that the intraperitoneal administration of 400 mg/kg L-DOPA to mice led to a 63% reduction in 5-HT content in the brain [Everett and Borcherding, 1970].

Implication for modulation of PFC Although DA is the most potent endogenous ligand known to activate the DRD4, it can also be activated by NE at submicromolar concentrations [Lanau et al., 1997, Newman-Tancredi et al., 1997]. While the affinity of the DRD4 for NE is at least five- to ten-fold lower than its affinity for DA [Oak et al., 2000], NE has a higher affinity for the D4 receptor than for any of the adrenergic receptors [Arnsten and Li, 2005]. The DRD4 has therefore also been referred to as a catecholamine receptor [Arnsten and Li, 2005]. Since NE terminals are present in the PFC, this suggests that L-DOPA administration might have two non-dissociable effects on the DRD4 in the PFC: one direct effect via increasing DA levels and an indirect effect via increasing NE levels.

4.6.5 Combining fMRI with neuropharmacological modulation

Given the unclear relative impact of DRD4 stimulation on the activity of different brain structures (vStr and PFC), it might be interesting to run a follow-up neuroimaging experiment using the same gambling task, polymorphism and a pharmacological approach similar or equal to the one described in this chapter.
However, there are some important caveats to be considered when combining neuropharmacological modulation with neuroimaging experiments that rely on the BOLD (blood oxygen level dependent)-signal or $H_2^{15}O$-PET as measures of rCBF. DAergic drugs are known to have vasoactive properties and may have direct effects on measures of rCBF. It has been shown that the vascular tree in prefrontal cortical areas of rhesus monkeys is directly innervated by DAergic afferents [Krimer et al., 1998]. A cholinergic vasodilatative system originating in the rat medial septal nucleus has also been shown [Sato et al., 2001] and activation of nicotinic receptors has been reported to cause an increase in cortical [Uchida et al., 1997] and hippocampal rCBF [Kagitani et al., 2000]. 5-HT might play a similar role given its vasoconstrictory affect via the 5-HT_{1B} receptor [5-HT_{1B} agonists (triptans) are used in the treatment of migraine headache, which is hypothesised to result from a vasodilation of cranial blood vessels].
Central to this issue is the question whether these vasoactive properties are *independent* of any vasodilation due to the increased metabolic demands after neuronal activation. For example, if a phasic DA release increases the activity of a given post-synaptic neuron and in doing so increases local rCBF, this were not a major problem because the increased rCBF then reflects an increase in activity of the post-synaptic neuron. However, all the studies mentioned [Krimer et al., 1998, Sato et al., 2001, Kagitani et al., 2000, Uchida et al., 1997] have controlled for metabolic effects and blood pressure [Sato et al., 2001] and still found vasodilatatory effects mediated by the cholinergic and DAergic system suggesting that the release of certain neurotransmitters may affect rCBF in ways that are independent of the neuronal metabolic process.
However, most of the fMRI designs are relatively protected from the *tonic* vasoactive effects of psychotropic drugs for two reasons. First, the modelling uses a high-pass filter that removes the effects of slow drifts in the BOLD signal. Second, one identifies regionally specific foci of differential activation. These foci are likely smaller than the region of monoaminergic or cholinergic vascular innervation.
In the future, more emphasis should be placed on PET tracer studies [*e.g.* using

a recently developed tracer that is highly selective for the DRD4[1], Prante et al., 2008] in the context of decision making experiments because only these studies may answer some of the questions mentioned above.

4.6.6 Does one gene determine one behaviour?

It has been pointed out already in the eighties that genes do not stand in a simple unidirectional relationship with behaviour [Pfaff, 1989]. The relationship between the one-dimensional simplicity of the genome (20'000 − 25'000 genes) and the three-dimensional complexity of the CNS is clearly not straightforward. It was suggested that the *one gene/one enzyme* hypothesis can in no way become a *one gene/one synapse* hypothesis let alone a *one gene/one behaviour* hypothesis [Changeux et al., 1998]. The action of many genes may "converge" on a given brain structure, and a single gene may have "divergent" effects on several different structures [Changeux, 1983].

An important issue in this context is the observation that the development of the CNS is guided by temporally and spatially regulated expression of proteins suggesting that some genes and proteins may influence CNS organisation only during specific phases of its development. For example Gorski et al. [2003] investigated the *in vivo* requirements for brain derived neurotrophic factors (BDNF) during development by generating an early-onset forebrain-specific BDNF mutant mice. Although these mice completely lacked BDNF in the forebrain during embryogenesis, they were healthy and no loss of specific cortical excitatory or inhibitory neurons was detected at birth. However, the neocortex of 5 wk old mice was thinner, which was attributable at least partly to neuronal shrinkage suggesting that BDNF plays a general role in supporting neuronal survival.

A recent study has shown that the valine allele of the BDNF valine to methionine substitution (Val(66)Met) polymorphism was associated with significantly higher mean neuroticism scores on the *NEO-Five Factor Inventory* in healthy subjects [Sen et al., 2003]. In light of the fact that BDNF is a universal neurotrophic factor supporting neuronal growth in the CNS in many species [Zigmond et al., 1999], it seems particularly difficult to provide *any* mechanism by which the BDNF Val(66)Met polymorphism might affect behaviour.

There is evidence to suggest that this developmental issue might be relevant for the DRD4 polymorphism as well. For example, Durston et al. [2005] reported that the average prefrontal gray matter volume is partially determined by the absence

---

[1] 2-[4-(4-(2-^{18}F-ethoxy)phenyl)piperazin-1-ylmethyl]pyrazolo[1,5-a]pyridine

versus presence of the 7R allele. Therefore, one could speculate that the DRD4 might play a regulatory role in the neuronal growth of prefrontal cortical inhibitory interneurons, on which the receptor is expressed (see also section 4.6.2). This sheds a different light on the relationship between DA and its impact on the DRD4 in adults. This issue is also important for the development of drugs which selectively bind to the DRD4 and which might be relevant for the treatment of certain DRD4-related psychiatric diseases.

Implications for pharmacogenetic studies Given the hypothetical impact of the DRD4 polymorphism on brain development [Durston et al., 2005], the polymorphism may therefore be associated with a phenotype (*e.g.* ADHD) that rather results from differences in brain morphology than from a difference in signal transmission at the DRD4. A novel drug for the treatment of *e.g.* ADHD in adults may therefore erroneously be informed by genetic association studies pointing towards the DRD4 as a potential target for drug action. However, if a drug (*e.g.* olanzapine) is used that binds specifically to the DRD4 and shows a DRD4 polymorphism dependent effect on a certain behaviour or disease symptom, it may be assumed that this in fact results from differences in signal transmission at the DRD4 and not from general differences in CNS development. However, this argument is exclusively valid for DRD4 selective compounds and not for *e.g.* L-DOPA, because of its lack of specificity for the DRD4. A general increase in CNS DA availability stimulates several types of DA receptors and their density and number may partly be determined by regional brain volume in turn. Therefore, L-DOPA administration may lead to behavioural effects that are conditional on the DRD4 polymorphism but these differential effects may have their origin in the difference in brain morphology. In summary, a pharmacogenetic approach to investigate behaviour or to treat psychiatric diseases should use a drug that is specific for the receptor polymorphism under investigation [but see Cohen et al., 2007]. Likewise, a more precise model of a gene-behaviour relationship can be established.

4.6.7 Implications for clinical practice in psychiatry

Pharmacogenetics has been proclaimed as a way of using genetic information in medicine in general to improve patient outcome. One of the areas where these techniques are likely to be applied in the future is in the pharmacotherapy of psychiatric disorders ["personalised psychiatry", see Morley and Hall, 2004]. While pharmacogenetics has the potential to positively impact on the treatment of psychiatric conditions, its use also raises some ethical and economic issues.

Treatment of Parkinson's disease

In this chapter, we show first evidence for a genotype dependent effect of anti-Parkinsonian medication on gambling behaviour. At first glance these results suggest that a subgroup of subjects might be vulnerable to pathological gambling. However, our experimental design does not allow making assertions about the general population of Parkinson's disease patients that suffers from pathological gambling. We used healthy male students as subjects and a task that has not been tested for external validity with respect to pathological gambling (as opposed to the *South Oaks Gambling Task*) [Lesieur and Blume, 1987] (but see section 5.5.1 on page 93). Moreover, we cannot draw conclusions from these results about a single individuum, since we have aggregate data at hand here. Most critically, however, the present data do not inform about the behavioural addiction process that might underlie pathological gambling. The investigation of the development of addiction processes in a controlled laboratory environment is for ethical reasons unfeasible in humans. Therefore, human addiction research is restricted to transsectional or longitudinal studies of individuals that are already addicted or become addicted during the study (*e.g.* pathological gamblers).

Therefore, the results presented here can only be viewed as a first hint for further studies investigating genetic risk factors for pathological gambling in Parkinson's disease patients. A number of questions have to be answered before it is worthwhile to bring genotyping of candidate genes such as the DRD4 gene into clinical routine in the pharmacotherapy of Parkinson's disease. These may include the following:

1. How does gambling behaviour relate to L-DOPA treatment and DRD4 genotype in Parkinson's disease patients?

2. What other polymorphisms contribute to the same phenotype?

3. How does this relationship depend on disease severity/ stage?

4. What is the influence of patients' sex?

5. Is there a drug dose – addiction severity relationship?

A hypothetical scenario   To get a glimpse into future issues that may arise in this context, we shall look at the following hypothetical scenario. Let's assume that we had initiated a longitudinal study with a sample of 250 Parkinson's disease patients not suffering from pathological gambling. Results show that within 1 y after the initiation of L-DOPA therapy, six out of a 100 patients who carry a 7R

4.6. Comments on Study 2

allele had developed pathological gambling, but only three of all the 4R carriers. Carrying a 7R allele thus triples the risk of suffering from pathological gambling in these patients. We therefore consider new strategies for clinical practice in the treatment of Parkinson's disease.

Personalised treatment: costs and benefits To assess whether genotyping could potentially help to improve drug therapy in Parkinson's disease patients, a coarse qualitative cost/benefit analysis will be given here. Some of the common costs of pathological gambling include financial hardship (via debts and asset losses) that may lead to legal consequences, such as bankruptcy, loans, or criminal acts to gain money [Ladouceur et al., 1994]. Costs imposed on the society by pathological gambling include the cost of crimes committed by some individuals and costs related to their treatment. Interpersonal problems between gamblers and their significant others include domestic violence, relationship breakdown, neglect of family, and may cause secondary costs due to the negative impact on the physical and mental health of family members [Raylu and Oei, 2002].

A personalised treatment also bears costs. As part of the preventive strategy, psychiatrists/ neurologists have to warn patients of the potential risk of developing the gambling disorder due to DAergic drug treatment. They should be informed about this fact *before* initiation of drug treatment [Voon et al., 2007a]. Moreover, drug administration should be monitored more carefully by the physician in subjects at risk, since an escalation of drug self-administration is often observed concomitantly with the onset of pathological gambling [Voon et al., 2007b]. Such provisions are relatively inexpensive, yet they might be effective.

On the other hand, insurance companies have to decide whether they are willing to bear costs associated with the new treatment strategy. They will view pre-therapeutic genotyping only as economic if the costs for genotyping and personalised treatment by the physician are offset by savings from avoiding the costs of treating patients. The financial damage to an individual that suffers from pathological gambling (see above) will not have to be covered by the insurance. However, this does not apply to the costs that arise for the treatment of health problems arising secondary to the gambling disorder. These secondary costs will be imposed on the insurance company and will likely be higher than those for genotyping and personalised treatment. Therefore, insurance companies have a clear incentive to support or request pre-therapeutic genotyping of Parkinson's disease patients in the future.

Based on the results of the hypothetical study mentioned above, we now decide to employ the devised strategy for the treatment of all Parkinson's disease patients who carry a 7R allele. We therefore treat 6% of these 7R allele carriers correctly and 94% incorrectly. This seems to be rather inefficient. However, since pathological gambling has such a fatal impact on a patient's social and economical wellbeing, these costs are far outweighed by the relatively low costs of an adjustment of the treatment strategy in the 7R allele carriers after genotyping of all 250 Parkinson's disease patients. However, a pharmacogenetics based treatment of Parkinson's disease patients bears a number of ethical risks mainly for the patients but also for the society.

Patient discrimination Because individuals may suffer from discrimination, patient privacy is an important issue raised by the application of pharmacogenetic testing to clinical treatment [Morley and Hall, 2004]. Although genetic testing does not show whether a patient will suffer from pathological gambling, testing may result in a patient being labelled as a "high risk" individual. Such patients may suffer similar insurance or employment discrimination to those individuals identified as being at high risk of developing a genetic disease such as Huntington's disease [Morley and Hall, 2004]. Subject's access to certain medications might also be restricted, since it is possible that only certain medications interact with the DRD4 polymorphism to increase the risk for pathological gambling. Yet, these medications might be also the most effective in treating motor symptoms for certain patients.

Gene patenting In the context of ethics and genetics, a bothersome issue is the gene patenting laws. For example, the U.S. Patent Application No. 200-602-63359 is issued for the human DRD4 and includes all associated "cardiovascular disorders, gastrointestinal and liver diseases, haematological disorders, neurological disorders and respiratory diseases". Most critically, the "invention also features compounds which bind to and/or activate or inhibit the activity of DRD4 as well as pharmaceutical compositions comprising such compounds."
Patenting of genes incur large costs on behalf of science, economy and society. Genetic code is not simply a chemical substance, but rather a form of information with many different functions. Scientific research should not be constrained by a patent whose aim is to protect one commercial use, but in this case protects all potential uses that are somehow linked to the information contained in the gene. The monopolistic character of gene patents therefore impedes scientific progress. In case of the U.S. Patent No. 200-602-63359, it is possible that the patent holder will handicap research with the aim of developing more efficient ADHD medication.

4.6. Comments on Study 2

Moreover, patent holders may block access to genetic resources and will cause high costs in the health care system, which have to be raised for continuing research and development in medicine.

In principle, it is possible that the patent holders of the U.S. Patent No. 200-602-63359 could also assert their claim if future DRD4 genotype-based therapies for Parkinson's disease were to be employed. This sheds a different light on the hypothetical cost/ benefit analysis outlined above. It is questionable whether insurance companies are also willing to cover costs of the patent claims.

The dopamine hypothesis of ADHD: revision necessary?

It is generally hypothesised that the neurobiological basis of ADHD is a relative hypo-DAergic state and is based on numerous findings, including observations of reduced volume of DAergic brain structures (*e.g.* smaller caudate nucleus and globus pallidus in ADHD subjects compared to control groups) [Swanson et al., 2007] and the observation that administering methylphenidate (MPH) leads to a reduction of ADHD symptomatology. MPH is an amphetamine that inhibits DA-reuptake by binding to the dopamine transporter (DAT) and thereby increases synaptic availability of DA. The hypothesis is further supported by genetic association studies showing that genes related to the DAergic system may play a role in ADHD [Faraone et al., 2005] with most consistent associations being reported for the DAT gene and the DRD4 gene [Roman et al., 2001, Li et al., 2006].

However, the DA deficit hypothesis of ADHD has recently been challenged [Gonon, 2009]. For example, it has been shown that atomoxetine, which exclusively binds and inhibits the norepinephrine transporter (NET), is also an effective treatment of ADHD. Furthermore, it has long been known that MPH also binds to the NET although with a somewhat lower affinity [Gatley et al., 1996, Kuczenski and Segal, 1997]. Finally, the question arises whether L-DOPA that effectively treats the DAergic deficits in Parkinson's disease patients is also effective to treat ADHD.

The data presented in here suggest that DAergic stimulation is associated with an increased propensity to gamble in subjects who carry at least one 7R allele. If an increased gambling propensity can be viewed as a form of poor inhibitory control (which is the primordial symptom of ADHD) it is surprising that L-DOPA administration did not lead to a *reduction* in gambling propensity in the 7R allele carriers.

Since we did not check whether ADHD symptomatology was present in our subjects, we have to be cautious in drawing conclusions about populations of ADHD affected individuals. Interestingly, however, previous studies showed that L-DOPA treatment of ADHD is not effective in treating symptoms [Overtoom et al., 2003]. Future studies should more closely investigate whether the differences in signal transduction at the DRD4 are partly responsible for ADHD using D4 selective agonists/antagonists (see also 4.6.6).

Chapter 5

Study 3: Prejudice and truth: the effect of testosterone administration on bargaining behaviour

5.1 Contributions

Experimental design was done by Ernst Fehr and me. Data collection and data analysis for the study presented in this chapter were done by me. Ernst Fehr coauthored the paper that resulted from this study. The comments on this study were written by me (section 5.5).

5.2 Introduction and results

TE is a steroid hormone, which is secreted in mammals by male testes and, to a much lesser extent, the female ovaries. TE is present in the CNS throughout life and affects brain development and sexual behaviour. In rodents, TE administration leads to substantial increases in aggressive behaviours [Beeman, 1947, Edwards, 1969]. Folk wisdom generalises and adapts these findings to humans, suggesting that TE induces antisocial, egoistic, or even aggressive behaviours [Bjorkqvist et al., 1994, Booth et al., 2006]. In fact, this "wisdom" has even reached the courtrooms because steroid induced rage has been used as legitimate defence in the United States [Pope and Katz, 1990]. As we will document below, the folk wisdom also strongly affected the subjects in our study because most of them believed in the folk hypothesis.

There is indeed evidence suggesting a link between TE and antisocial behaviour in humans [Dabbs et al., 1995, Dabbs and Hargrove, 1997]. In a sample of 692 adult male prisoners, for example, those who had a history of rape, murder, and armed robbery had higher salivary TE levels than those who had only a history of theft and drug abuse [Dabbs et al., 1995]. According to disciplinary records, those inmates with relatively higher TE levels were reported to be more involved in overt confrontations in prison and more likely to violate prison rules compared to those with relatively lower levels. A similar pattern was observed in a study comprising 87 female prison inmates [Dabbs and Hargrove, 1997].

While these facts are consistent with the folk hypothesis, they do not constitute convincing evidence for two reasons. First, the evidence is purely correlative and does not show that TE is causally involved in generating the observed behaviours. Second, the alternative hypothesis proposing that TE plays an important role in status-related behaviours in human social interaction can also explain the norm violating behaviours [Mazur and Booth, 1998, Mazur, 2005, Josephs et al., 2003, 2006, Schultheiss et al., 1999, Rowe et al., 2004]. According to this hypothesis, TE induces status-seeking and leadership in situations that constitute a potential challenge to a person's status. Thus, in settings such as prisons, where rigid social hierarchies impose subordinate positions on individuals, those who are predisposed to seek leadership and status may question the hierarchy in antisocial and rebellious ways [Mazur and Booth, 1998, Booth et al., 2006]. Thus, the folk hypothesis and the status hypothesis make identical predictions in these situations.

While the status hypothesis constitutes a plausible alternative to the folk hypothesis, it unfortunately remains largely based on correlative evidence [Mazur and Booth, 1998, Mazur, 2005, Josephs et al., 2003, 2006, Schultheiss et al., 1999, Rowe et al., 2004]. However, a rigorous separation of the two hypotheses is possible because TE-induced leadership and status seeking may take a prosocial dimension if the prosocial behaviour enables individuals to master a social challenge or to secure their leadership. Thus, the task is to generate an experimental situation where the folk hypothesis predicts antisocial behaviour while the status hypothesis predicts prosocial behaviour.

The *Ultimatum Game* [Gueth et al., 1982] represents such a situation because previous evidence [Camerer, 2003, Knoch et al., 2006b] indicates the existence of a strong fairness norm in this game. Thus, subjects can behave prosocially in this game by obeying the norm or they can behave antisocially by violating it. We therefore examined the impact of exogenously administered TE and placebo on the

5.2. Introduction and results

propensity to obey or violate the fairness norm in this game.
Real money is at stake in the *Ultimatum Game*; two parties, A and B, have to agree on the division of 10 money units (MUs). Party A, often referred to as the proposer, is in a kind of leadership position because only she can propose how the 10 MUs will be allocated between A and B. Party B, often referred to as the responder, is in the weaker position because B can only accept or reject A's proposal, but cannot make a counteroffer. Thus, A has the power to stipulate an ultimatum to B, which gave the game its name. If B accepts A's proposal, the proposed allocation will be implemented. Party B can also reject A's proposal, however; in this case, neither party earns anything.

This bargaining game is ideal for our purposes because many studies [Camerer, 2003, Knoch et al., 2006b] indicate that player B perceives low bargaining offers as unfair, while the equal split is the salient fairness norm in this situation. As a consequence, many subjects in the role of B reject low offers, meaning that neither player earns anything. From the viewpoint of the folk hypothesis, the question is therefore whether the administration of TE increases the frequency of low offers. In the context of our experiment, low offers constitute an unambiguous violation of a prevailing normative standard and can thus be viewed as a form of antisocial behaviour. Low offers can be considered antisocial, not just due to the fact that they violate a fairness norm, but also because they bear the increased risk of social conflict (*i.e.* a rejection), meaning that both players may ultimately end up with zero earnings. Thus, the folk hypothesis unambiguously predicts that TE leads to more unfair offers.

The status hypothesis proposes that subjects who receive TE will place a higher value on status than subjects with placebo. Previous evidence suggests that this impact of TE on status concerns is most likely to occur in situations in which subjects' status is potentially challenged [Mazur and Booth, 1998, Josephs et al., 2003, 2006, Archer, 2006]. This is exactly the situation of a proposer in the *Ultimatum Game*, who has the power to make the offer and thus can influence the subsequent course of action. The proposer can assert her leadership by achieving mutual cooperation (*i.e.*, by inducing the responder to accept the offer), or she can risk the denial of leadership by making an unfairly low offer. Thus, because the risk of rejection implies a denial of leadership, subjects who place a high value on status gain more from an acceptance compared to those placing a low value on status. Therefore, if TE increases status concerns, we should observe fairer offers among subjects who received TE. In a double-blind, placebo-controlled study design a total of 60 women participated in our experiment in the role of a proposer. All of them were required to not take contraceptives, had a regular menstrual cycle and were in the early follicular phase of the cycle, when the endogenous level of sex steroids tends to be low and stable. Every subject played three independent *Ultimatum Games* with three different responders. To avoid having the experience of acceptances or rejections affect the proposers' behaviour, they did not receive feedback about their responders' actions until the end of the experiment. In each game, the proposer could offer the responder 0, 2, 3 or 5 MUs (out of 10 MUs). 0.5 mg of TE or placebo was applied sublingually 4 h before subjects played the *Ultimatum Game*. This is a well established procedure [Tuiten et al., 2000] that has reliably shown to generate behavioural effects [van Honk et al., 2001, 2005]. We recruited only women because the parameters (quantity and time course) for inducing neurophysiological effects after a single sublingual administration of 0.5 mg of TE are known in women [Tuiten et al., 2000], whereas these parameters are unknown in men. In order to check whether subjects noticed the substance they had been given, we also asked them whether they believed they received placebo or TE. Their beliefs were unrelated to the actual substance they received (Mann-Whitney test, $P = 0.208$, n = 60, two-tailed), indicating that they did not know what they had been given. However, even though subjects did not know whether they received placebo or TE, it is important to control for the possible influence of their beliefs because TE is probably one of the most widely discussed hormones in the popular press and, therefore, it is possible that prior knowledge about TE might affect their behaviour [Bjorkqvist et al., 1994]. Ethical concerns require researchers to inform subjects that they will either receive a placebo or TE, and the prior knowledge about TE may pollute a possible impact of TE on behaviour. In particular, subjects' behaviour may be affected by their belief in the folk hypothesis. A survey that we conducted several months after the experiment confirmed subjects' strong beliefs in the folk hypothesis: they believed that TE increases contentious, selfish and aggressive behaviour. 52% of them even spontaneously mentioned the word "aggressive" when asked to indicate how TE administration affects the behaviour of individuals. We also gave subjects a list of paired behavioural or intentional attributes such as "aggressive - peaceful". The subjects then could express their views about whether TE makes people strongly aggressive, weakly aggressive, weakly peaceful, strongly peaceful or neither aggressive nor peaceful". 80% of the subjects expressed the view that TE makes people strongly or weakly aggressive. The list of paired attributes also contained words such as contentious and selfish. 83% agreed that TE makes people more contentious and roughly 50% thought that it makes them more selfish (only 5% thought that it makes them less selfish). In view of these strong subjective be-

5.2. Introduction and results

liefs in the folk hypothesis, we controlled for subjects' beliefs about whether they had received TE or placebo in our statistical analysis. In addition, we always controlled for repeated measurements by taking each subjects' average offer across the three *Ultimatum Games* as the unit of observation.

The folk hypothesis predicts that proposers with TE make lower offers. In contrast to this prediction, subjects who received TE actually made significantly higher offers (ANOVA, main effect of TE, $F = 5.78$, $P = 0.020$, $n = 60$), with placebo subjects offering on average 3.40 MUs, while subjects with TE offered 3.90 MUs [Figure 5.1 (**A**)]. Thus, while we find no support for the folk hypothesis, our results are consistent with the status hypothesis. However, we also find strong support for a "belief effect". Subjects who merely believed that they have received TE make much lower offers than those who believed they received placebo [Figure 5.1 (**B**); ANOVA, main effect of believed TE, $F = 8.97$, $P = 0.004$, $n = 60$]. Interestingly, if we control simultaneously for both the belief and the TE effects the belief effect is even larger than the actual TE effect. The belief effect reduces offers by 0.92 MU while the pure TE effect increases offers by 0.64 MUs. No interaction effect between TE and believed TE is observed (ANOVA, interaction between TE and believed TE, $F = 0.90$, $P = 0.346$, $n = 60$).

Interestingly, the belief effect is present regardless of whether subjects actually

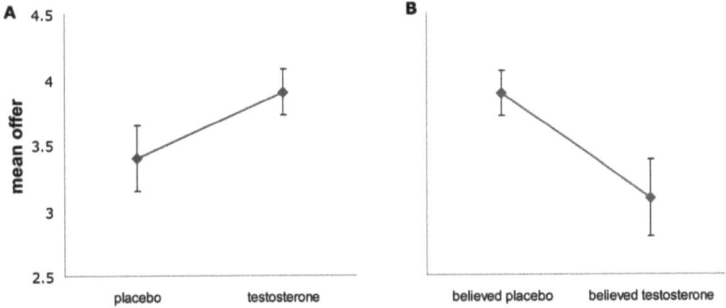

Figure 5.1: The proposers' mean offers across treatments and beliefs. (**A**) Mean offers in the placebo and the TE group. Subjects who received TE make significantly fairer offers. (**B**) Mean offers for the subjects who believed that they received placebo compared to those subjects who believed that they received TE. Subjects who believed that they received TE make much more unfair offers. Error bars indicate SEM.

received TE or whether they actually received placebo. Among the subjects who were randomly assigned to the placebo group, those who believed that they received placebo offered on average 3.66 MU, and 51% of the offers were even at the maximum of 5 MU [Figure 5.2 (**A**)]. This result is in sharp contrast with the offers of those who actually received placebo but believed they received TE. These subjects make extremely low average offers of 2.37 MU; only 10.5% of the offers were at the maximum of 5 MU, while 53% of the offers were only 2 MU. We are not aware of any other study that reports such low offers in the *Ultimatum Game*. Even the proposers in the society with the lowest offer in the cross-cultural study of Henrich et al. [2005] offered a higher average share (26%) to the responder [Henrich et al., 2005]. A similar belief effect is present in those subjects who were randomly assigned to the TE group. The average offer in the group that actually received TE and believed they received TE was 0.67 MU lower than in the group that received TE and believed they received placebo [Figure 5.2 (**B**)].

The pure TE effect is present regardless of subjects' beliefs. If we exclusively anal-

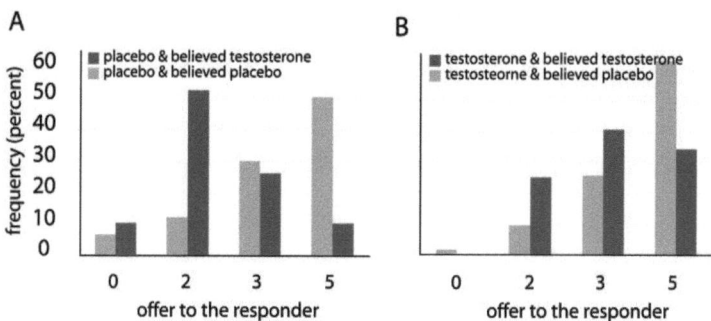

Figure 5.2: Distribution of proposers' offers conditional on their beliefs. (**A**) Distribution of offers for subjects who received placebo. Among these subjects, those who believed that they received TE (red bars) make much more unfair offers compared to those who believed that they received placebo (blue bars). (**B**) Distribution of offers for subjects who received TE. A similar pattern prevails among these subjects: those who believed that they received TE (red bars) make more unfair offers compared to those who believed that they received placebo (blue bars). In both graphs, the modal choice for those who believed that they received placebo is the fair split, *i.e.*, an offer of 5, while the modal offer is below 5 for those who believed that they received TE.

5.2. Introduction and results

yse data from subjects who believed that they received placebo [Figure 5.3 (**A**)], we find that those who actually received TE made relatively high average offers of 4.11 MU, with 63% of all offers at the maximum. In contrast, those who actually received placebo made offers that were 0.45 MU lower and only 51% of the offers were equal to the maximal offer. We observe an even stronger effect among those who believe they received TE [Figure 5.3 (**B**)]. Those who believe they received TE but actually received placebo offered only 2.37 MU, while those who share the same belief but actually received TE offered 3.43 MU on average. This TE effect is also visible in the salient rightwards shift of the distribution of offers depicted in Figure 5.3 (**B**).

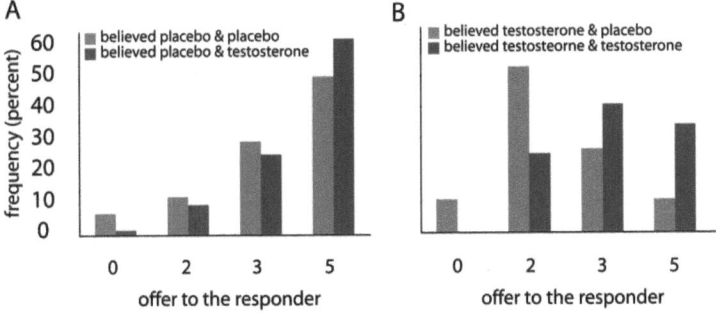

Figure 5.3: Distribution of proposers' offers across the placebo and the TE group. (**A**) Distribution of offers for subjects who believed that they received placebo. Among these subjects, those who received TE (violet bars) made more fair offers compared to those who received placebo (green bars). (**B**) Distribution of offers for subjects who believed that they received TE. A similar pattern prevails among these subjects: those who received TE (violet bars) made much fairer offers than those who received placebo (green bars).

5.3 Discussion

Taken together, these results cast strong doubt on the folk hypothesis and are consistent with the status hypothesis. However, higher offers among the subjects with TE could also be due to a possible impact of TE on subjects' mood or anxiety. For this reason, we controlled for potential indirect effects of TE in several ways (see section 5.4). We measured subjects' mood, their calmness, and their wakefulness immediately after substance administration and again 4 h later, immediately before they made their decisions in the *Ultimatum Game*. Immediately after the administration of TE or placebo, the two groups were identical in all these dimensions (Mann-Whitney tests: wakefulness $P = 0.941$, mood $P = 0.863$, calmness $P = 0.287$, $n = 60$, two-tailed). There were also no differences between the TE and the placebo group immediately before playing the *Ultimatum Game* (Mann-Whitney tests: wakefulness $P = 0.365$, mood $P = 0.157$, calmness $P = 0.411$, $n = 60$, two-tailed). We also measured changes between the first and the second measurement and found no differences (Mann-Whitney tests: wakefulness $P = 0.760$, mood $P = 0.328$, calmness $P = 0.732$, $n = 60$, two-tailed). These results indicate that TE neither influenced subjects' mood and arousal; nor did it affect changes in these variables throughout the experiment. Therefore, the higher prevalence of fair offers in the TE group cannot be attributed to indirect effects operating via these variables.

Perhaps our finding that TE increases fair bargaining behaviour can be attributed to the effects of TE on anger or anxiety. Or maybe our randomisation did not work perfectly and there were trait differences across the treatments in subjects' propensity to feel anger and anxiety. To address these questions, we measured subjects' propensity to feel anger or anxiety (trait anger and trait anxiety, respectively), at the beginning of the experimental session. We found no significant differences between the TE and placebo group (Mann-Whitney tests: trait anger: $P = 0.402$, trait anxiety: $P = 0.807$, $n = 60$, two-tailed). Moreover, it is a priori rather unlikely that TE increased fair behaviour due to an increase in subjects' anxiety or fear because the literature points in the opposite direction. If anything, TE may have a fear and anxiety reducing effect [van Honk et al., 2005, Aikey et al., 2002]; and a lower fear of being rejected should lead to a decrease in *Ultimatum Game* offers. However, we nevertheless examined this question more thoroughly and thus measured subjects' actual feelings of anxiety (state anxiety) and anger (state anger) immediately after substance administration, and 4 h later, immediately before they played the *Ultimatum Game*. Again, there are no significant differences between the placebo group and the TE group. Neither after substance administration (Mann-Whitney tests: state anger: $P = 0.788$, state anxiety: $P = 0.528$, $n = 60$, two-tailed) nor

5.3. Discussion

before the beginning of the *Ultimatum Game* (Mann-Whitney tests, state anxiety: $P = 1.000$; state anger: $P = 0.615$, $n = 60$, two-tailed) are there differences across treatment groups, nor is there a treatment difference in the changes of these variables between the two time points of the measurements (Mann-Whitney tests: state anger: $P = 0.637$, state anxiety: $P = 0.339$, $n = 60$, two-tailed).

In principle, TE application could also have had indirect effects via moderating CORT levels in our subjects. An androgen based down regulation of the HPA axis has been discussed in the literature [Viau, 2002]. To address this issue, we repeatedly measured subjects' salivary CORT levels as a reliable and valid measure of HPA axis activity [Kirschbaum and Hellhammer, 1994]; these measures were taken before the administration of TE and before the subjects played the *Ultimatum Game*. We find no significant difference across the two treatment groups at either time of CORT measurements (Mann-Whitney tests: before TE administration $P = 0.726$, before playing the *Ultimatum Game* $P = 0.960$, $n = 58$; two-tailed), nor do we observe any differences in CORT changes between the two measures (Mann-Whitney test, $P = 0.546$). Thus, there are no differences in CORT levels and CORT changes across the TE and placebo group.

Another interesting question concerns the potential role of endogenous baseline TE levels in our experiment. If subjects in the TE group exhibited higher baseline TE levels, one could argue that the difference in baseline TE levels causes the effect on proposers' offers and not the exogenous administration per se. For this reason, we measured salivary TE levels immediately before the substance administration. We find no significant difference in baseline TE levels in the two treatment groups (Mann-Whitney test: $P = 0.739$, $n = 59$, two-tailed). Furthermore, we also controlled for a potential impact of baseline TE at the individual subject level by controlling for baseline levels in an ANOVA of the offers. This analysis again confirms that TE administration also increases proposers' offers if we control for baseline TE (ANOVA, main effect of TE, controlled for baseline TE values, $F = 6.21$, $P = 0.016$), and the impact of baseline TE on proposers' offers is insignificant (ANOVA, main effect of baseline TE values, $F = 1.09$, $P = 0.362$, $N = 59$). Finally, we checked whether the effect of exogenous TE on proposer behaviour is a function of baseline TE levels in the sense that subjects with low endogenous baseline levels react particularly strongly to the exogenous administration of TE. However, the interaction effect between endogenous TE levels and the exogenous TE administration on proposers' offers is also insignificant (ANOVA, $F = 1.13$, $P = 0.345$, $n = 59$). Thus, these results unambiguously show that endogenous baseline TE levels cannot explain the higher prevalence of fair offers. Rather, it is the experimental administration of TE that caused the higher bargaining offers.

The fact that TE enhances aggression in some animals and the broad media coverage of results suggesting a relationship between endogenous TE-levels and antisocial behaviour has led public opinion to believe that TE may generally cause antisocial, selfish and aggressive behaviours. However, our results cast serious doubt on the folk hypothesis because subjects with exogenously administered TE make much fairer offers in the bargaining game. The increase in fair bargaining behaviour among subjects with TE also led to a higher acceptance rate (ANOVA, $F = 4.18$, $P = 0.046$, $n = 60$), thereby reducing bargaining conflicts and increasing the efficiency of social interactions. Indirect effects of TE on mood, arousal, anxiety, anger or stress cannot explain these results. We also observe that the endogenous TE level does not affect behaviour or the effect of TE on behaviour in our setting. Thus, we can conclude that TE administration causes an increase in fair bargaining offers in our subjects. This result is consistent with the status hypothesis [Mazur and Booth, 1998, Mazur, 2005, Josephs et al., 2003, 2006, Schultheiss et al., 1999] which proposes that subjects with TE care more for their status, which in turn increases the utility loss associated with rejections. It is also worthwhile to point out that if the status hypothesis is correct, then TE subjects do not comply with the fairness norm because they value fairness *per se* but because norm compliance helps them to assert their status and their leadership role.

The impact of TE on compliance with the fairness norm in our setting supports the view that biological factors play an important role in human social interaction [Mazur and Booth, 1998, Mazur, 2005, Josephs et al., 2003, 2006, Schultheiss et al., 1999, Kosfeld et al., 2005]. This does, of course, not mean that psychological factors are not important. In fact, our finding that subjects' beliefs about TE are powerful predictors of behaviour in the bargaining game points towards the importance of psychological and social factors. This finding also teaches an important methodological lesson for future studies: it is crucial to control for subjects' beliefs because the pure substance effect may be otherwise under- or overestimated. Thus, it is important to keep an eye on biological and socio-psychological factors in human social interaction for substantive and for methodological reasons.

5.4 Methods

5.4.1 Subjects

Sixty-two healthy women (mean age ± SD: 25.3 ± 6.20 years) participated in the study after providing written informed consent to the study; the local ethics committee had previously approved it. Only women were recruited because the parameters (quantity and time course) for inducing neurophysiological effects after a single sublingual administration of 0.5 mg of TE are known in women [Tuiten et al., 2000], whereas these parameters are unknown in men. Before admission to the study, all subjects were screened in a telephone interview to exclude medication intake, somatic diseases, or any neurological or psychiatric disorders. They were further instructed to abstain from alcohol or caffeine intake and smoking 24 h before the experiment. Additionally, only subjects who did not use hormonal contraceptives participated in the study and all of them were checked for having a regular menstrual cycle. Moreover, we conducted a pregnancy test before the beginning of the experiment, to preclude pregnancy. Subjects were all invited to the experiment within 10 d after the beginning of the menstrual cycle, when endogenous levels of sex hormones tend to be low and stable. A physician was at the experimenter's disposal during the course of the whole experiment. Two subjects were excluded from the analysis because they had an overall score of 2 SD above the mean in the global severity index of the *Symptom Checklist* for psychopathological symptoms [Derogatis, 1977].

5.4.2 Experimental procedure

All experiments took place at the experimental laboratory of the Institute for Empirical Research in Economics, where a total of ten sessions were conducted. All sessions started at 1.00 pm and lasted approximately 5 h. Following oral instructions at the beginning of each session, subjects were randomly assigned to the TE or placebo group (double-blind, placebo-controlled study design). They received one single dose of TE or placebo, sublingually. Due to the established time lag of 4 h for behavioural effects to appear after sublingual application of 0.5 mg TE in young, healthy women [Tuiten et al., 2000, van Honk et al., 2001, 2005], a long waiting period was an integral part of our study. During this period, our subjects were required to stay in the laboratory room and read newspapers. This was to ensure that no social interaction outside the laboratory took place.
The TE preparation contained 0.5 mg of TE base with hydroxy-propyl-β-cyclodextrin

as a carrier [Stuenkel et al., 1991]. The placebo contained no TE but was otherwise identical. Both preparations were manufactured by Laboswiss, in Davos, Switzerland. The *Ultimatum Game* is played with two types of players, a proposer and a responder, who have to agree on the division of 10 MUs. The proposer can decide upon the distribution of the 10 MUs. In our experiment, the proposer could propose an offer of 5, 3, 2, or 0 MUs to the responder. This ensured a clear separation between an offer that is regarded as fair (5 MUs) and offers that are perceived as unfair (3, 2 or 0 MUs). The responder then had to either accept or reject this proposal. If the responder accepted the proposer's offer, the proposed allocation was implemented. However, the responder could also reject the proposal; in this case neither party earned anything.

Subjects were randomly and anonymously assigned to the role of either the proposer or the responder and did not know the identity of the persons with whom they were matched in the experiment. After subjects read the instructions (they are available from the authors upon request), we checked whether they had understood the payoff structure by having them complete several control questions. All subjects answered these control questions correctly. In addition, we summarised the experimental procedure orally. In the experiment, every proposer made three propositions on the distribution of MUs while paired with three different randomly selected interaction partners. No pair of subjects interacted twice. The proposer did not receive feedback about the responders' choices until the end of the experiment. All decisions in the *Ultimatum Game* were implemented in zTree software and presented on computer screens [Fischbacher, 2007]. Subjects received a base fee of one hundred Swiss francs for participation in the experiment. Each MU in the *Ultimatum Game* was worth one Swiss franc. Each subject received her earnings consisting of the base fee plus the earned MUs in private at the end of the experiment.

5.4.3 Salivary measurements

We measured salivary TE concentrations before administration of 0.5 mg of sublingual TE or placebo. We deliberately measured salivary TE levels because taking blood is highly invasive and could induce stress in subjects. Salivary TE has proven to be a reliable measure of the biologically active, non-protein bound proportion ("free TE") of TE in blood serum. Before sublingual application of either TE or placebo, mean ($\pm$ SD) baseline salivary TE concentration was 38.51 pg/ml ($\pm$ 38.83 pg/ml) in the group randomly assigned to receive the placebo and 38.68 pg/ml ($\pm$ 34.85 pg/ml) in the group randomly assigned to receive TE. We additionally analysed salivary CORT levels before TE or placebo administration and immediately before the *Ultimatum Game* was played. Before administration of TE or placebo, salivary CORT concentrations were 10.60 nmol/l (± 6.11 nmol/l) in the placebo group and 10.00 nmol/l (± 5.10 nmol/l) in the TE group. Before the *Ultimatum Game* was played, salivary CORT concentrations were 4.96 nmol/l (± 3.19 nmol/l) in the placebo group and 4.72 nmol/l (± 2.59 nmol/l) in the TE group. We used the IBL SaliCaps Kit (IBL-Hamburg, Hamburg, Germany) for saliva specimen collection; subjects were requested to transfer 1 ml of saliva into the test tubes, which were then immediately frozen at -80 C. Saliva analysis was performed by IBL-Hamburg (Germany) using commercially available chemiluminescence-immunoassay with an intra- and inter-assay coefficient of variation lower than 10%.

5.4.4 Questionnaires

The validated German versions of the following questionnaires were included: The 90-item Symptom Checklist (revised version) [Derogatis, 1977], the *Multidimensional Mood Questionnaire* [Steyer et al., 1997], the State-Trait Anxiety Inventory [Laux, 1981], and the *State-Trait Anger Expression Inventory* [Schwenkmezger et al., 1992]. Psychological well-being was assessed at the beginning of the experiment by the *90-item Symptom Checklist* (revised version). This is a multidimensional self-report instrument designed to screen for a broad range of psychological problems and symptoms of psychopathology. The inventory contains a total of ninety items, each of which is rated on a 5-point scale indicating the degree of distress associated with each symptom [Derogatis, 1977]. The global severity index is calculated from the sum of all ratings divided by the number of rated items. This global severity index forced the exclusion of two subjects from the analysis, due to an overall score of 2 SD above the mean. We assessed the treatment group subjects believed themselves to be in by asking them at the end of the experiment whether they believed they received TE or placebo.

We measured mood and arousal at the beginning of the study and immediately before the *Ultimatum Game* (*i.e.*, 4 h after substance administration) by means of the *Multidimensional Mood Questionnaire* (MDBF) . The MDBF consists of three subscales, termed elevated vs. depressive mood, wakefulness vs. sleepiness, and calmness vs. restlessness. Subjects rate these items on a 5-step scale ranging from 1 (not at all) to 5 (very strongly). Subscale scores are calculated by summing up the respective item ratings [Steyer et al., 1997].

Anxiety was measured by the *State-Trait Anxiety Inventory* [Laux, 1981]. The inventory is measured by a 40-item self-rated psychometric instrument. The state-trait anxiety measure consists of items rated on four-point intensity scales (1 = not at all; 2 = somewhat; 3 = moderately; 4 = very much). Trait anxiety was assessed at the beginning of the experiment, while state anxiety was assessed immediately after the administration of the substance and before the start of the *Ultimatum Game*. State anxiety denotes a transitory emotional state characterised by subjective feelings of tension and apprehension. Trait anxiety indicates individual differences in anxiety proneness and refers to a general tendency to respond to perceived threats in the environment with anxiety.

Anger was measured by the *State-Trait Anger Expression Inventory* [Schwenkmezger et al., 1992]. The inventory is measured by a 20-item self-rated psychometric instrument. The state and trait anger measure consists of items rated on four-point intensity scales (1 = not at all; 2 = somewhat; 3 = moderately; 4 = very much). Trait anger was again assessed at the beginning of the experiment, and the state measure was assessed twice, once immediately after the substance administration and once at the beginning of the behavioural task. State anger denotes the intensity of angry feelings experienced "right now, at this moment". Trait anger represents individual differences in general proneness to react angrily in anger provoking situations.

5.4.5 Statistical analysis

Statistical analysis is based on non-parametric Mann-Whitney tests and ANOVA. All tests are two-tailed tests. We examined the impact of TE [with a binary indicator for TE indicating whether the subject received TE (= 1) or placebo (= 0)], the impact of belief about TE administration [(with a binary indicator for subjects who believed they received TE (= 1) or placebo (= 0)], the impact of baseline levels of salivary TE (we grouped subjects into four equally sized groups), and the impact of the interactions between these variables in a univariate one-way ANOVA on proposers' offers in the *Ultimatum Game*.

5.4.6 *Post-hoc* online survey

All subjects that participated in the experiment in *Chapter 5* were approached by email and asked whether they would be willing to participate in the survey. They were informed that they will receive an Amazon gift-certificate upon answering all questions. 92% of all subjects participated. The survey was structured as follows: first, subjects were asked how TE administration would modify any given person's

5.4. Methods

behaviour. They were asked to answer this question without the aid of class books or any other information material. Second, they were asked whether they expect the administration of TE would modify their behaviour if they were to receive it (see Table 5.1). Third, they were given a list of 13 two-poled opposed items, where they could indicate the expected behaviour modification after application of TE ranging from "none", "weak behaviour modification" to "strong behaviour modification" (see Table 5.2).

Table 5.1: Items subjects spontaneously mentioned are listed in the left column. The middle column shows the percentage of subjects who mentioned the respective item at least once. The right column shows the percentage of subjects who indicated that the effect would also appear if they were to receive TE.

Items	Percentage	Percentage(self)
aggressive	56%	68%
risk seeking	25%	78%
dominant	2%	0%
interested in sex	5%	100%
self confident	20%	64%
mood changes	20%	64%
other behaviours	33%	72%
biological effects	18%	60%
no change	2%	100%
drive	10%	80%
goal oriented	5%	33%
egoistic	3%	50%

Table 5.2: Subjective ratings of the believed effects of TE administration. Pairs of the two opposed-poled items are listed in the left and right columns. The average ratings (± SD) of 55 subjects are indicated (1 = change towards left item, 5 = change towards right item).

Left pole	Average rating	± SD	Right pole
diffident	4.35	0.68	laddish
aggressive	1.70	0.84	peaceful
risk seeking	1.63	0.88	risk averse
dominant	1.78	0.69	submissive
distrustful	2.97	0.67	trustful
generous	3.19	0.62	greedy
fearful	4.13	0.67	fearless
awake	2.5	0.86	tired
dizzy	3.33	0.78	clear-thinking
egoistic	2.19	0.78	altruistic
manly	1.78	0.74	less manly
competitive	1.69	0.78	less competitive
self-confident	1.89	0.79	insecure

5.5 Further comments on Study 3

Summary of main findings We found that sublingual administration of 0.5 mg of TE to 60 female proposers playing a one-shot and anonymous *Ultimatum Game* was associated with an increase in fair offers compared to placebo administration. Moreover, those subjects who believed to have received TE made substantially lower offers compared to those who believed to have received placebo. The TE effect on proposer offers was significant in an ANOVA controlled for the TE believed treatment group. The effect of the believed TE treatment group was also significant. In the following, these findings will be discussed in two different parts. The first part discusses the obtained findings on the level of content. Alternative explanations for the observed effect of TE on proposer offers as well as additional control experiments will be suggested. Furthermore, data on the responder behaviour will be provided and discussed in the context of status. The discussion of status will be closed by providing a potential further TE administration experiment investigating competitive behaviour in the laboratory. Subsequently, a critical discussion of the external validity of experimental economic paradigms and neuroeconomic experiments will be provided with reference to the findings presented in this chapter.

The second part discusses the neuroendocrinological aspects of TE administration experiments. More specifically, the relative specificity of TE administration effects on the androgen system will be discussed. Moreover, the role of the enzyme aromatase, which metabolises TE into E2, in mediating TE administration effects will be looked at more closely. Furthermore, because the employed methodological approach leads to supraphysiological TE serum levels, the potential inhibitory feedback responses on the level of the HPG-axis will be discussed. Each section closes with a discussion of potential control experiments.

5.5.1 External validity of economic games

One critique experimental economics often face is that of their low external validity of their experiments due to the high degree of artificiality [Loewenstein, 1999]. Artificiality often implies experimental control, however, and therefore increases internal validity. External validity refers to the ability to generalise from the research context to the settings that the research is intended to approximate. Internal validity refers to the ability to draw confident conclusions from one's research. The design of an experiment is therefore always directed by a trade-off between the demands for high internal as well as external validity.

For example, we recruited only female subjects for the experiment in this chapter and one might criticise the subject pool bias. The question that arises here is whether we can extend the findings that TE administration increases the frequency of fair proposer offers also to men. Moreover, it is important to know whether some sort of selection bias was present in the group of female subjects that volunteered for the experiment described here. One might assume that they differ with respect to anxiety, since ingesting TE is not a usual thing to do for women. A t-test indeed revealed that trait anxiety scores on the *State-Trait Anxiety Inventory* [Laux, 1981] of the present sample of females were significantly higher than those of a sample of females who volunteered for a regular experiment ($P < 0.01$). Therefore, women who were willing to ingest TE had significantly lower trait anxiety scores. This in itself would not be a problem. However, if subjects with higher trait anxiety experienced an anxiolytic effect of TE, this might not be true for subjects with lower trait anxiety. This potential confound decreases the external validity of the experiment presented in this chapter. Furthermore, subjects were mostly university students from Switzerland and it were interesting to see whether TE administration had a different effect given to subjects who have a different cultural background [see *e.g.* Henrich et al., 2005]. Moreover, the money the subjects won in the *Ultimatum Game* was only a small fraction of the overall payment and resulting in incentive dilution. Finally, some subjects had participated in similar experiments before, while others did not. One might therefore criticise that we used a heterogeneous subject pool of inexperienced and experienced individuals.

While the artificiality of anonymous laboratory tasks is also an attempt to remove context effects, this is often difficult to accomplish. It has to be assumed that experimental subjects are engaged in a constant search for cues about how they are supposed to behave [Loewenstein, 1999]. A relevant study in this context is the one performed by [Hoffman et al., 1994], in which the authors investigated the influence of environmental cues on proposer behaviour in the *Dictator Game* (see section 1). Proposers who were given detailed instructions about the elaborate measures that had been taken to ensure anonymity gave away less money than in conditions that did not ensure such a high degree of anonymity. The authors conclude that "people act as if they are other regarding because they are better off with the resulting reputation. Only under conditions of social isolation are these reputation concerns of little force".

However, if human complex decision making processes are to be investigated in a well controlled environment, this has to be performed in a laboratory. Experimental economics offers a way to investigate complex decision making processes in the laboratory at the cost of having a relatively low external validity. One has therefore

5.5. Comments on Study 3

to be cautious in drawing conclusions directly from the laboratory into the real world.

The combination of these paradigms with neurobiological methods may, however, increase the external validity of the measure derived in a certain paradigm since the combination allows us to draw a more fine-grained picture of the processes that underlie human decision making. Because the knowledge of these neurobiological processes could potentially also inform us about the underlying motives that drive decision making in a particular paradigm, this will inform us about the type of external environment to which the findings can be extended.

For example, a recent twin-study reported that trusting behaviour measured by the *Trust Game* has a heritable component [Cesarini et al., 2008]. Since one can assume that genetic behavioural traits are stable, the very aspect of *Trust Game* behaviour that has proven to be heritable must have an external analogue. It is unlikely that an individual's genetic makeup will uniquely predict *Trust Game* behaviour, but not other, related behaviours outside the laboratory.

In a recent experiment, we could show that baseline cortical activity in the right DLPFC predicts individual risk-taking behaviour in the laboratory [Gianotti et al., 2009]. Baseline cortical activity was measured using resting-state EEG and a source-localisation technique before subjects performed the risk-taking task. Individuals with higher baseline cortical activity in the right DLPFC brain area displayed more risk aversion than did other individuals. Given that resting-state EEG has been reported to capture stable individual differences in neural activity [Kondacs and Szab, 1999], this finding demonstrates that neural characteristics reminiscent of a psychological trait variable may partially predict highly complex behaviours such as risky decision making. As in the example described above, it is unlikely that this relatively stable neurophysiological measure will only predict behaviour in the laboratory.

In other cases, decision making paradigms have been externally validated directly. For example, the gambling task applied in *Chapter 4* has been successfully used to predict children's behaviour in real-world traffic. Those who were classified as risk takers by the gambling task made more crossing decisions at a busy one-way street than risk avoiders and tolerated shorter time intervals between initiation of the crossing decision and arrival of the next vehicle [Hoffrage et al., 2003].

5.5.2 Testosterone rules...?

An issue that often comes up in personal discussions (especially between women and men) is how much influence hormones have on our everyday life. The rodent literature reviewed in section 2.3.3 suggests a strong influence of TE on socially aggressive behaviour. On the other hand it has been suggested that one of TE's role in primate behaviour is to support non-aggressive dominance behaviour, which has taken the form of ritualised demonstrations of power, rather than actual physical fights resulting in injuries [Mazur, 1985, Mazur and Booth, 1998]. Therefore the role of TE in primate behaviour is much more complex than in rodents. These differences have been accounted for by the relatively greater influence of the neocortex in guiding behaviour in primates as opposed to rodents [Mazur and Booth, 1998]. It has been hypothesised that the non-isometric brain expansion observed throughout primate evolution might be due to the cognitive demands of the increasingly complex social worlds these animals live in [Dunbar, 1992, 1998]. While parts of the brain (such as the neocortex) concerned with higher-order cognitive capacities get bigger across phylogenies, those parts of the brain involved in regulating the hormonal control of primary motivated behaviours have become relatively smaller (*e.g.* hypothalamus and the preoptic area) [Keverne et al., 1996]. It has therefore been speculated that human social behaviour differs from that of animals in that it is relatively liberated from the constraints of the hormonal state [Curley and Keverne, 2005]. Thus, TE's effect on human social behaviour may be strongly moderated by intrapsychic, social, and cultural factors and may be less unidirectional than in rodents [Christiansen, 2001].

Given the relatively strong manipulation of serum TE levels achieved by the procedure presented in this chapter [see also Figure 5.4 below and Tuiten et al., 2002], it is intriguing that it did neither affect subjects self-reports of anxiety, anger nor other mental states (wakefulness, restlessness and mood). It is worth noting that no study has yet reported an effect of a single dose of TE on consciously perceived emotions or mental states in women [Tuiten et al., 2002, van Honk et al., 2001, 2004, 2005, van Honk and Schutter, 2007, Hermans et al., 2006a,b, 2008]. Nevertheless, most of these studies reported behavioural effects, which are mostly considered to be generated outside of conscious awareness (*e.g.* Emotional Stroop Task effects using subliminally presented angry facial expressions, subtle autonomic arousal responses and reduced startle effects). In summary, although it appears that TE has effects on everyday human behaviour, these are likely not consciously noticeable. It has been argued that this is due to the fact that TE acts mostly on subcortical structures, whose size is relatively small compared to the neocortex.

The question whether TE "rules" our lives can only be answered on a qualitative level. The limited number of TE administration studies suggest that TE administration in humans has anxiety (but not fear) reducing effects, increases libido

[Christiansen, 2001], facilitates autonomic arousal in response to the presentation of angry faces as well as decreases recognition of emotional facial expressions [Tuiten et al., 2002, van Honk et al., 2001, 2004, 2005, van Honk and Schutter, 2007, Hermans et al., 2006a,b, 2008].

5.5.3 Specificity of testosterone effects

Throughout this chapter, the term "TE *administration* causes" was used to refer to the causal role of TE in modulating social decision making behaviour. The term "TE administration" refers to *any* process, that is initiated by the application of TE and does not imply that TE is the major agent that causes the effects. Unfortunately, it also precludes to make conclusions about the role of the hormone TE *per se* in the reported effects. A deeper insight into the role of the androgen system in social decision making behaviour is only possible if the pharmacological methodology is refined.

Is testosterone a *pro*hormone?

The idea that TE may act as a prohormone in mediating certain behavioural processes (*i.e.* TE has to be metabolised into an active form with respect to the process) is partly based on the early observations that not TE, but rather E2 is the substance that defeminises the CNS in the developing mammalian fetus [Zigmond et al., 1999]. As outlined in section 2.3.1 on page 20, the two major pathways of TE metabolism involve the formation of two neuroactive steroids, DHT and E2. While DHT is a classical androgen, which has a high affinity for the AR (see page 21), E2 activates its own receptor system (ER-α and ER-β). These metabolic pathways are mediated by 5α-reductase (DHT) and aromatase (E2), respectively.

There is direct evidence from pharmacokinetic trials showing that sublingual TE administration leads to elevated DHT and E2 levels. For example, the pharmacokinetic study (see section 2.3.1) performed by Stuenkel et al. [1991] reported the following: serum TE concentration increased 63-fold compared to baseline ($\pm$ 24.2 SEM) 20 min after sublingual application of 5.0 mg of TE. Critically, serum levels of DHT and E2 increased 9-fold ($\pm$ 1.3) and one-fold ($\pm$ 0.4), respectively. For DHT, t_{max} was reached after $\approx$ 30 min and for E2, t_{max} was reached after $\approx$ 120 min. Although this study was performed in hypogonadal males, it provides direct evidence that elevated levels of neuroactive metabolites of TE are observed in blood serum after TE administration.

5.5.4 Suppression of the reproductive axis

Besides the unclear source of TE administration effects, the procedure we and others [*e.g.* Tuiten et al., 2002, van Honk et al., 2001, 2004, 2005, van Honk and Schutter, 2007, Hermans et al., 2006a,b, 2008] used give rise to a number of additional limitations.

First, all studies used a dose of 0.5 mg of TE applied sublingually, resulting in unphysiologically high levels of TE [ten-fold increased levels compared to baseline as reported by Tuiten et al., 2002].

We attempted to replicate these findings in a small pharmacokinetic study in which we administered our own TE preparation (manufactured by Laboswiss, Davos, Switzerland) to eight healthy women. Serum TE concentrations were measured once before TE administration and 15, 30 and 60 min after administration. The results of this study are shown in Figure 5.4. Mean (± SEM) baseline concentrations were 0.47 ng/ml (± 0.07), t_{max} was reached 15 min after TE administration with a corresponding maximum concentration (c_{max}) of 1.85 ng/ml (± 0.37). Thus, the sublingual application of TE resulted in an almost 400% increase in serum TE concentration relative to baseline. While t_{max} is equal, c_{max} is lower than the one reported previously [estimated from Figure 2.3: 6 ng/ml; Tuiten et al., 2002]. Such high levels likely induce a negative feed-back response on GnRH and LH release at the hypothalamic and pituitary level, respectively.

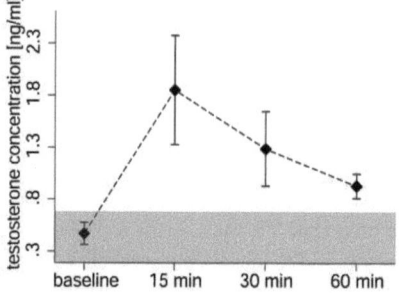

Figure 5.4: Pharmacokinetics of serum TE after administration of a single dose of 0.5 mg of sublingual TE with a HP-β-CD carrier to eight healthy females (manufactured by Laboswiss, Davos, Switzerland). The shaded area indicates the normal physiological range of serum TE concentration in healthy young females.

LH is released in an episodic or pulsatile fashion from the pituitary gland and the pulsatile secretion of LH seems to be a result of episodic hypothalamic discharge of GnRH into the portal vein and subsequent stimulation of the pituitary [Santen and Bardin, 1973]. Under physiological conditions, serum LH levels are kept within a tight range, reflecting the balance between stimulation by GnRH and inhibition by gonadal sex steroids [Karsch, 1987]. The negative feedback control of LH se-

5.5. Comments on Study 3

cretion is mediated primarily by E2 [Karsch, 1987]. LH secretion reacts sensitive to elevated concentrations of E2 in women [Karsch, 1987] and since we can expect substantial conversion of TE into E2 in the hypothalamus (see section 5.5.3), TE administration might have affected GnRH and therefore LH secretion. Changes in one hormonal axis are expected to affect other systems, which will then interfere with the behavioural measure. For example, if GnRH and LH pulsatility is changed, this should lead to a changed secretion of estrogens and androgens from the ovaries in female subjects (see section 2.3.2). Unfortunately, we did not measure LH and GnRH in the pharmacokinetic study described above, but future pharmacokinetic studies investigating E2 and TE administration effects should determine these important parameters.

Second, because the sublingual administration interferes with the measurement, salivary TE levels cannot be determined to verify the resulting rise in serum levels of TE. Salivary steroid concentrations can easily be determined and correlate well with the ones obtained from serum measurements [Riad-Fahmy et al., 1987, Granger et al., 2004]. This approach has been used in a wealth of studies (see section 5.4.3 and page 88). Female salivary TE concentrations range from 5 to 50 pg/ml and its detection requires sensitive immuno-assays. However, after *sublingual* application of 0.5 mg of TE these results may be confounded substantially by traces of TE base remaining in the mouth giving yield to shifted measures. In fact, if only 0.0001% of the administered amount of TE is retained in the oral mucosa, salivary TE concentrations measured thereafter would be twice as high as those that are usually detected under normal conditions. Blood-sampling may avoid this confound, however, the use of syringes could interfere with the behavioural measure due to psychological stress of the subjects Kirschbaum and Hellhammer [1994] (see also page 25).

Third, relevant amounts of E2 are secreted from the ovary already 3 d after beginning of menstruation [Nieschlag, 2006], which could affect behaviour, *e.g.* by priming or additive effects. Furthermore, GnRH release and LH secretion responds differently to E2 at different points in the menstrual cycle [Karsch, 1987].

There are possible solutions for the draw-backs mentioned in the sections above. Since the negative hypothalamic feed-back response to exogenous TE seems to be less sensitive in men compared to women [Nieschlag, 2006], a potential way to achieve methodological improvements is to use male subjects. Moreover, a different TE administration procedure could be used. TE is available in a cutaneous formulation for men (approved for the treatment of male hypogonadism; Androgel ®), which is easy to apply and should not interfere with TE measurements in saliva. Finally, a reliable inhibition of aromatase using exemestane is potentially more effective in male subjects, since they secrete E2 in lower and more stable concentrations [Weinbauer et al., 2000].

Part III

General conclusions

Neuroeconomics has recently emerged as an interdisciplinary effort to bridge the gap between neuroscience and economic theories and methodology. Although many argue that the flow of information between the two sub-disciplines is unidirectional, neuroeconomics has challenged both standard economic theory and improved the understanding of human individual and social decision making from a neurobiological perspective. Past studies investigating the neurobiological aspects of decision making primarily reported correlative data; relatively few investigated the causal contribution of a given neurobiological system to decision making. The main goal of the present thesis was to investigate whether human individual and social decision making can be modulated using neuromodulatory approaches.

Central to neuroeconomic experiments is the use of monetary incentives to quantify how much an individual subjectively values an outcome of a chosen option. These options are usually presented in the form of experimental economics paradigms involving one decision maker or many simultaneously interacting decision makers. The neuroeconomic studies presented in this thesis were performed in a well-controlled laboratory environment, which is essential for the investigation of the neurobiological aspects underlying individual and, in particular, social decision making.

With respect to individual decision making, the present thesis reports data on the role of the anti-Parkinsonian drug L-DOPA in gambling behaviour. Using an intuitively comprehensible gambling task, we were able to show that L-DOPA administration caused an increase in gambling behaviour, conditional on a subjects' DRD4 genotype. More specifically, we could show that DAergic stimulation in healthy humans is associated with an increased propensity to gamble in subjects who carry a risk allele, the 7R allele of the DRD4 polymorphism, for impulse control related disorders such as ADHD and pathological gambling. These findings are the first to show a pharmacogenetic effect on risky decision making, emphasising the importance of including genetic information in neuropharmacological intervention studies investigating behaviour in the laboratory. While we can speculate about the contribution of different brain structures in the modulation of gambling behaviour based on the neuroanatomical distribution of the DRD4, future neuroimaging studies may provide a more detailed answer. fMRI and $H_2^{15}O$-PET are seductive approaches for achieving this; these methods have to used with caution, however. Many pharmacological compounds are known to be vasoactive and may therefore interfere with rCBF in ways that are independent of the vasodilatative effects observed as part of the neuronal metabolic process. A more elaborate way to investigate the distribution and role of the DRD4 in the human brain is to use receptor specific radioligands in PET. A further option is the use of EEG, which has proven to be a sensitive measure in neuropharmacological studies.

We have suggested that the reported pharmacogenetic effect on gambling behaviour may have important implications for the treatment of Parkinson's disease patients, since pathological gambling is increasingly reported as a side-effect of DAergic drug treatment in these patients. Because pathological gambling is regarded as a behavioural addiction process, which is for obvious reasons not amenable to scientific inquiry in the laboratory, a number of questions remain open. Moreover, the neurophysiological interactions of L-DOPA administration with the DRD4 polymorphism probably differ in healthy subjects compared to patients affected with Parkinson's disease. However, if future association studies should find a statistical relationship between certain polymorphisms such as the DRD4 polymorphism and pathological gambling in medicated Parkinson's disease patients, genotyping might become part of clinical practice in the treatment of these patients. This will raise important ethical questions, including those of patient discrimination by insurance companies and those with respect to gene patent claims.

Concerning social decision making, the thesis shows evidence that social decision making may be influenced by the well known hormone TE. Using the *Ultimatum Game*, we were able to show that TE administration is associated with an increased frequency of fair proposer offers. This finding contrasts with the impact of subjects' beliefs about the TE treatment: those who believed they received TE made remarkably lower offers compared to those who believed they received placebo. These findings show for the first time that people's beliefs about TE and its actual behavioural effects diverge dramatically and overhaul the traditional view that TE is the cause of violence. The influence of the popular view about well-known substances such as TE should receive particular attention in future studies investigating social decision making. While we suggest that the actual effect of TE is a manifestation of its impact on status seeking behaviour, a number of issues remain unanswered, on the methodological level, on the neuroendocrinological level, as well as with regards to content. With respect to the latter, additional experiments have to be performed to investigate whether TE administration in females in fact does not cause prosocial behaviour *per se*. To further corroborate the status hypothesis, future experiments should also investigate concepts which are closely related to status, such as competitiveness and reputation formation.

In a further step, it should be investigated whether the effects reported are restricted to females or if they also appear in males. Given that men have relatively higher TE levels than women who have higher E2 levels in turn, it were interesting to see whether these hormones fulfill the same or different roles in either sex with respect to social decision making. Neuroendocrinological studies in rodents, non-human primates, and humans suggest an important role of the enzyme aromatase in this context. The enzyme converts TE to E2 and there is much reason to believe that many effects we observe after TE administration in fact result from its conversion to E2. This enzyme can be inhibited pharmacologically and future experiments should elucidate whether this inhibition can abolish TE effects or not. Recent PET evidence in non-human primates suggests that aromatase is mainly located in the amygdala, which is an important structure in regulating socio-emotional behaviours. Therefore, a preliminary hypothesis is that TE administration exerts its effects on social decision making via an E2-mediated modulation of the amygdala. From a methodological viewpoint, the sublingual administration of 0.5 mg TE to women has many disadvantages. Although it results in a reliable increase in serum TE levels within several min, the levels achieved are in the supraphysiological range and likely result in a negative feed-back response on the level of the hypothalamus resulting in a decreased secretion of LH and GnRH. These hypothalamic hormones may then affect other hormonal systems giving rise to a confound. Moreover, the sublingual application precludes the measurement of sex hormones in saliva. A potential way to achieve improvements in this context is to use a transcutaneous TE administration procedure that allows for a convenient measurement of the achieved TE levels in saliva. Moreover, the transcutaneous TE formulation has an advantageous pharmacokinetic profile: serum levels are more stable and better controllable.

In summary, the present thesis shows experimental evidence that complex decision making processes may be modulated on the neurochemical and on the neuroendocrinological level. Furthermore, the data presented here suggest that neurostimulation is a promising approach for modulating decision making on the neuroanatomical level. These levels are clearly not independent, however, they all constitute experimental points of contact for investigating the causal role of neurobiological systems in modulating human decision making. The ethical issues that arise when performing studies using neuromodulatory methods have to be considered carefully. In all studies presented in this thesis each subject participated voluntarily and on the basis of the provision of all relevant information. The experimental nature of the intended procedure was made clear at the outset, and all participants were fully informed of any reasonably foreseeable risks or discomforts. Moreover, they were informed about the fact that they would not derive any direct benefit from their participation in the study. However, the findings presented in this thesis may have potential applications for a variety of psychiatric and neurological diseases such as addiction, depression and Parkinson's disease. Since these are often characterised by impaired decision making behaviour, the present experiments may also contribute to a better understanding of these diseases. Finally, the studies presented in this thesis may contribute to the development of new theories and study designs in neuroendocrinology, neuropharmacology, neuroeconomics, and social neuroscience.

Part IV

Appendix

Appendix

List of abbreviations

^{11}C L-DOPA	^{11}C labelled L-DOPA PET tracer	65
^{18}F L-DOPA	^{18}F labelled L-DOPA PET tracer	65
17-β-HSD	17-β-hydroxysteroid dehydrogenase	20
5-HT	5-hydroxy tryptamine or serotonin	11
5-HTP	5-hydroxy tryptophan	11
5-HTTPP	Serotonin transporter polymorphism	15
7R allele	7 repeats allele	13
AADC	Aromatic amino-acid decarboxylase	11
ACC	Anterior cingulate cortex	10
ACTH	Adrenocorticotropic hormone	20
ADH	Aldehyd-dehydrogenase	11
ADHD	Attention deficit hyperactivity disorder	14
ANOVA	Analysis of variance	40
AR	Androgen receptor	21
BA	Brodmann area	7
BBB	Blood brain barrier	11
BDNF	Brain derived neurotrophic factor	70
BOLD signal	Blood-oxygen level dependent signal	69
c_{max}	Maximum serum or salivary concentration	98
cAMP	Cyclic adenosine-monophosphate	12
CNS	Central nervous system	22
COMT	Catechol-O-methyl transferase	11
CORT	Cortisol	23
CRH	Corticotropin releasing hormone	23
CSF	Cerebrospinal fluid	11
DA	Dopamine	4
DAT	Dopamine transporter	75

List of abbreviations

DAT polym.	DAT 40 base-pair VNTR polymorphism	67
DBH	Dopamine-β-hydroxylase	11
DHEA	Dihydroepiandrosterone	20
DHT	Dihydrotestosterone	20
DLPFC	Dorsolateral prefrontal cortex	6
DNA	Desoxynucleic acid	21
DOPAC	Dihydroxyphenylacetic acid	11
DRD2 polym.	Taq1A DA receptor D2 polymorphism	15
DRD4 polym.	DA receptor D4 VNTR polymorphism	13
E2	17-β-estradiol	20
EEG	Electroencephalography	7
ER-α	Estrogen receptor alpha	21
ER-β	Estrogen receptor beta	21
fMRI	Functional magnetic resonance imaging	7
FSH	Follicle stimulating hormone	24
FWHM	Full-width at half-maximum	37
G_i	Inhibitory G-protein	12
G_s	Stimulatory G-protein	12
GABA	Gamma-aminobutyric acid	12
GIRK channel	G-protein coupled inward rectifying potassium channel	13
GnRH	Gonadotropin releasing hormone	24
H$_2$^{15}O	^{15}O labelled H$_2$O PET tracer	8
HP-β-CD	Hydroxy-propyl-β-cyclodextrin	22
HPA axis	Hypothalamic-pituitary-adrenal axis	23
HPG	Hypothalamic-pituitary-gonadal axis	23
HVA	4-hydroxy-3-methoxyphenylacetic acid/ homovanillic acid	11
L-DOPA	L-dihydroxphenylalanine	4
LH	Luteinising hormone	24
LTD	Long-term depression	45
MDBF	Multidimensional mood questionnaire	89
MPH	Methylphenidate	75
MS	Magnetic stimulation	52
MT	Motor threshold	10
NE	Norepinephrine	11
NET	Norepinephrine transporter	75

List of abbreviations

OFC	Orbitofrontal cortex	5
PET	Positron emission tomography	7
PFC	Prefrontal cortex	5
rCBF	Regional cerebral blood flow	8
ROI	Region of interest	39
SD	Standard deviation	37
SEM	Standard error of the mean	24
SHBG	Sex hormone binding globuline	21
SPM	Statistical parametric mapping	39
t_{max}	Time of maximum plasma or saliva concentration	22
TE	Testosterone	4
TH	Tyrosine hydroxylase	11
TMS	Transcranial magnetic stimulation	4
TrpH	Tryptophan hydroxylase	11
VAS	Visual analogue scale	57
VLPFC	Ventrolateral prefrontal cortex	5
VNTR	Variable number tandem repeat	13
VPA	Vaginal pulse amplitude	23
vStr	Ventral striatum	16

Bibliography

B. Abler, H. Walter, A. Wunderlich, J. Grothe, C. Schonfeldt-Lecuona, M. Spitzer, and U. Herwig. Side effects of transcranial magnetic stimulation biased task performance in a cognitive neuroscience study. *Brain Topogr*, 17(4):193–196, 2005.

G. E. Abraham. Ovarian and andrenal contribution to peripheral androgens during the menstrual cycle. *J Clin Endocrinol Metab*, 39:339–346, 1974.

R. F. Ackermann, D. M. Finch, T. L. Babb, and Jr. Engel, J. Increased glucose metabolism during long-duration recurrent inhibition of hippocampal pyramidal cells. *J Neurosci*, 4(1):251–264, 1984.

J. L. Aikey, J. G. Nyby, D. M. Anmuth, and P. J. James. Testosterone rapidly reduces anxiety in male house mice (mus musculus). *Horm Behav*, 42(4):448–460, 2002.

APA. *Diagnostic and statistical manual of mental disorders DSM-IV*. American Psychiatric Association, Washington, DC, 4th edition, 1995.

J. Archer. Testosterone and human aggression: an evaluation of the challenge hypothesis. *Neurosci Biobehav Rev*, 30(3):319–345, 2006.

A. F. T. Arnsten and B. M. Li. Neurobiology of executive functions: catecholamine influences on prefrontal cortical functions. *Biol Psychiatry*, 57:1377–1384, 2005.

A. R. Aron, P. C. Fletcher, E. T. Bullmore, B. J. Sahakian, and T. W. Robbins. Stop-signal inhibition disrupted by damage to right inferior frontal gyrus in humans. *Nat Neurosci*, 6(2):115–116, 2003.

V. Asghari, S. Sanyal, S. Buchwaldt, A. Paterson, V. Jovanovic, and H. H. M. Vantol. Modulation of intracellular cyclic-amp levels by different human dopamine d4 receptor variants. *J Neurochem*, 65(3):1157–1165, 1995.

T. Baumgartner, M. Heinrichs, A. Vonlanthen, U. Fischbacher, and E. Fehr. Oxytocin shapes the neural circuitry of trust and trust adaptation in humans. *Neuron*, 58:639–650, 2008.

E. A. Beeman. The relation of the interval between castration and 1st encounter to the aggressive behavior of mice. *Anat Rec*, 99(4):570–571, 1947.

H. M. Behre, K. Abshagen, M. Oettel, D. Huebler, and E. Nieschlag. Intramuscular injection of testosterone undecanoate for the treatment of male hypogonadism: phase i studies. *Eur J Endocrinol*, 140:414–419, 1999.

C. Bergh, T. Eklund, P. Sodersten, and C. Nordin. Altered dopamine function in pathological gambling. *Psychol Med*, 27(2):473–475, 1997.

N. Birbaumer and R. F. Schmidt. *Biologische Psychologie*. Springer Medizin Verlag, Heidelberg, 6., vollst. berarb. u. erg. aufl. edition, 2006.

M. Bixo, T. Baeckstroem, B. Winblad, and A. Andersson. Estradiol and testosterone in specific regions of the human female brain in different endocrine states. *J Steroid Biochem Mol Biol*, 55:297–303, 1995.

K. Bjorkqvist, T. Nygren, A. C. Bjorklund, and S. E. Bjorkqvist. Testosterone intake and aggressiveness - real effect or anticipation. *Aggr Behav*, 20(1):17–26, 1994.

K. J . Black and J.H. Friedman. Repetitive and impulsive behaviors in treated parkinson disease. *Neurology*, 67(7):1118–1119, 2006.

K. S. Blair, E. Finger, A. A. Marsh, J. Morton, K. Mondillo, B. Buzas, D. Goldman, W. C. Drevets, and R. J. R. Blair. The role of 5-httlpr in choosing the lesser of two evils, the better of two goods: examining the impact of 5-httlpr genotype and tryptophan depletion in object choice. *Psychopharmacology (Berl)*, 196(1):29–38, 2008.

F. E. Bloom, D. J. Kupfer, and B. S. Bunney. *Psychopharmacology the fourth generation of progress*. Raven Press, New York, NY, 1995.

A. Booth, D. A. Granger, A. Mazur, and K. T. Kivlighan. Testosterone and social behavior. *Soc Forces*, 85(1):167–191, 2006.

M. Brett, J.-L. Anton, R. Valabregue, and J.-B. Poline. Region of interest analysis using an spm toolbox. *Neuroimage*, 16(2):497, 2002.

F. Brighina, G. Giglia, S. Scalia, M. Francolini, A. Palermo, and B. Fierro. Facilitatory effects of 1 hz rtms in motor cortex of patients affected by migraine with aura. *Exp Brain Res*, 161(1):34–38, 2005.

BIBLIOGRAPHY

T. J. Brozoski, R. M. Brown, H. E. Rosvold, and P. S. Goldman. Cognitive deficit caused by regional depletion of dopamine in prefrontal cortex of rhesus-monkey. *Science*, 205(4409):929–932, 1979.

H. G. Burger and S. R. Davis. The role of androgen therapy. *Best Pract Res Clin Endocrinol Metab*, 16(3):383–393, 2002.

J. T. Cacioppo and G. G. Berntson. *Social neuroscience*. MIT press, Cambridge, M. A., 2002.

C. F. Camerer. *Behavioral game theory: experiments in strategic interaction*. Princeton University Press, Princeton, N.J., 2003.

J. J. Carmody. The birth of neuro-endocrinology: contemporary scientific blindness. 2008.

E. Cashdan. Hormones, sex, and status in women. *Horm Behav*, 29(3):354–366, 1995.

D. H. Catlin, C. K. Hatton, and S. H. Starcevic. Issues in detecting abuse of xenobiotic anabolic steroids and testosterone by analysis of athletes' urine. *Clin Chem*, 43(7):1280–1288, 1997.

D. Cesarini, C. D. Dawes, J. H. Fowler, M. Johannesson, P. Lichtenstein, and B. Wallace. Heritability of cooperative behavior in the trust game. *Proc Natl Acad Sci U S A*, 105(10):3721–3726, 2008.

J. P. Chalmers, R. J. Baldessarini, and R. J. Wurtman. Effects of l-dopa on norepinephrine metabolism in the brain. *Proc Natl Acad Sci U S A*, 68(3):662–666, 1971.

S. R. Chamberlain, U. Muller, A. D. Blackwell, L. Clark, T. W. Robbins, and B. J. Sahakian. Neurochemical modulation of response inhibition and probabilistic learning in humans. *Science*, 311(5762):861–863, 2006.

F. M. Chang, J. R. Kidd, K. J. Livak, A. J. Pakstis, and K. K. Kidd. The world-wide distribution of allele frequencies at the human dopamine d4 receptor locus. *Hum Genet*, 98(1):91–101, 1996.

J. P. Changeux. Concluding remarks: on the "singularity" of nerve cells and its ontogenesis. *Prog Brain Res*, 58:465–478, 1983.

J. P. Changeux, D. Bertrand, P. J. Corringer, S. Dehaene, S. Edelstein, C. Lna, N. Le Novre, L. Marubio, M. Picciotto, and M. Zoli. Brain nicotinic receptors: structure and regulation, role in learning and reinforcement. *Brain Res Brain Res Rev*, 26 (2-3):198–216, 1998.

R. Chen, J. Classen, C. Gerloff, P. Celnik, E. M. Wassermann, M. Hallett, and L. G. Cohen. Depression of motor cortex excitability by low-frequency transcranial magnetic stimulation. *Neurology*, 48(5):1398–1403, 1997.

D. R. Cherek, W. Schnapp, F. G. Moeller, and D. M. Dougherty. Laboratory measures of aggressive responding in male parolees with violent and nonviolent histories. *Aggr Behav*, 22(1):27–36, 1996.

C. L. Chio, R. F. Drong, D. T. Riley, G. S. Gill, J. L. Slightom, and R. M. Huff. D4 dopamine receptor-mediated signaling events determined in transfected chinese hamster ovary cells. *J Biol Chem*, 269(16):11813–11819, 1994.

P. A. Chouinard, Y. D. Van der Werf, G. Leonard, and T. Paus. Modulating neural networks with transcranial magnetic stimulation applied over the dorsal premotor and primary motor cortices. *J Neurophysiol*, 90(2):1071–1083, 2003.

K. Christiansen. Behavioural effects of androgen in men and women. *J Endocrinol*, 170(1):39–48, 2001.

B. Chung, K. J. Matteson, R. Voutilainen, T. K. Mohandas, and W. L. Miller. Human cholesterol side-chain cleavage enzyme, p450scc - cdna cloning, assignment of the gene to chromosome-15, and expression in the placenta. *Proc Natl Acad Sci U S A*, 83(23):8962–8966, 1986.

L. Clark, F. Manes, N. Antoun, B.J. Sahakian, and T. W. Robbins. The contributions of lesion laterality and lesion volume to decision-making impairment following frontal lobe damage. *Neuropsychologia*, 41(11):1474–1483, 2003.

C. R. Cloninger, T. R. Przybeck, and D. M. Svrakic. The tridimensional personality questionnaire: U.s. normative data. *Psychol Rep*, 69(3 Pt 1):1047–1057, 1991.

J. M. Coates and J. Herbert. Endogenous steroids and financial risk taking on a london trading floor. *Proc Natl Acad Sci U S A*, 105(16):6167–6172, 2008.

M. X. Cohen, A. Krohn-Grimberghe, C. E. Elger, and B. Weber. Dopamine gene predicts the brain's response to dopaminergic drug. *Eur J Neurosci*, 26(12):3652–3660, 2007.

BIBLIOGRAPHY

M. L. Collaer and M. Hines. Human behavioral sex differences: a role for gonadal hormones during early development? *Psychol Bull*, 118(1):55–107, 1995.

D. E. Comings, N. Gonzalez, S. J. Wu, R. Gade, D. Muhleman, G. Saucier, P. Johnson, R. Verde, R. J. Rosenthal, H. R. Lesieur, L. J. Rugle, W. B. Miller, and J. P. MacMurray. Studies of the 48 bp repeat polymorphism of the drd4 gene in impulsive, compulsive, addictive behaviours: Tourette syndrome, adhd, pathological gambling, and substance abuse. *Am J Med Genet*, 88(4):358–368, 1999.

E. Congdon, K. P. Lesch, and T. Canli. Analysis of drd4 and dat polymorphisms and behavioral inhibition in healthy adults: implications for impulsivity. *Am J Med Genet B Neuropsychiatr Genet*, 147B(1):27–32, 2008.

R. Cools. Role of dopamine in the motivational and cognitive control of behavior. *Neuroscientist*, 14(4):381–395, 2008.

R. Cools, L. Clark, A. M. Owen, and T. W. Robbins. Defining the neural mechanisms of probabilistic reversal learning using event-related functional magnetic resonance imaging. *J Neurosci*, 22(11):4563–4567, 2002.

R. Cools, R. A. Barker, B. J. Sahakian, and T. W. Robbins. L-dopa medication remediates cognitive inflexibility, but increases impulsivity in patients with parkinson's disease. *Neuropsychologia*, 41(11):1431–1441, 2003.

R. Cools, L. Altamirano, and M. D'Esposito. Reversal learning in parkinson's disease depends on medication status and outcome valence. *Neuropsychologia*, 44(10):1663–1673, 2006.

P. Corvol and C. W. Bardin. Species distribution of testosterone-binding globulin. *Biol Reprod*, 8(3):277–282, 1973.

J. F. Couse, D. O. Bunch, J. Lindzey, D. W. Schomberg, and K. S. Korach. Prevention of the polycystic ovarian phenotype and characterization of ovulatory capacity in the estrogen receptor-alpha knockout mouse. *Endocrinology*, 140(12):5855–5865, 1999.

J. P. Crean, H. de Wit, and J. B. Richards. Reward discounting as a measure of impulsive behavior in a psychiatric outpatient population. *Exp Clin Psychopharmacol*, 8(2):155–162, 2000.

H. D. Critchley, D. R. Corfield, M. P. Chandler, C. J. Mathias, and R. J. Dolan. Cerebral correlates of autonomic cardiovascular arousal: a functional neuroimaging investigation in humans. *J Physiol*, 523 Pt 1:259–270, 2000.

O. Curet, T. Dennis, and B. Scatton. The formation of deaminated metabolites of dopamine in the locus coeruleus depends upon noradrenergic neuronal activity. *Brain Res*, 335(2):297–301, 1985.

J. P. Curley and E. B. Keverne. Genes, brains and mammalian social bonds. *Trends Ecol Evol*, 20(10):561–567, 2005.

J. M. Dabbs. Age and seasonal-variation in serum testosterone concentration among men. *Chronobiol Int*, 7(3):245–249, 1990.

J. M. Dabbs and M. F. Hargrove. Age, testosterone, and behavior among female prison inmates. *Psychosom Med*, 59(5):477–480, 1997.

J. M. Dabbs, R. B. Ruback, R. L. Frady, C. H. Hopper, and D. S. Sgoutas. Saliva testosterone and criminal violence among women. *PAID*, 9(2):269–275, 1988.

J. M. Dabbs, B. C. Campbell, B. A. Gladue, A. R. Midgley, M. A. Navarro, G. F. Read, E. J. Susman, Lmjw Swinkels, and C. M. Worthman. Reliability of salivary testosterone measurements - a multicenter evaluation. *Clin Chem*, 41(11):1581–1584, 1995.

A. A. d'Alfonso, J. van Honk, E. Hermans, A. Postma, and E. H. de Haan. Laterality effects in selective attention to threat after repetitive transcranial magnetic stimulation at the prefrontal cortex in female subjects. *Neurosci Lett*, 280(3):195–198, 2000.

J. W. Dalley, T. D. Fryer, L. Brichard, E. S. J. Robinson, D. E. H. Theobald, K. Laane, Y. Pena, E. R. Murphy, Y. Shah, K. Probst, I. Abakumova, F. I. Aigbirhio, H. K. Richards, Y. Hong, J. C. Baron, B. J. Everitt, and T. W. Robbins. Nucleus accumbens d2/3 receptors predict trait impulsivity and cocaine reinforcement. *Science*, 315(5816):1267–1270, 2007.

A. R. Damasio. *Descartes' error, emotion, reason and the human brain.* Putnam, New York, NY, 1994.

Z. J. Daskalakis, B. Moller, B. K. Christensen, P. B. Fitzgerald, C. Gunraj, and R. Chen. The effects of repetitive transcranial magnetic stimulation on cortical inhibition in healthy human subjects. *Exp Brain Res*, 174(3):403–412, 2006.

S. R. Davis and H. G. Burger. The role of androgen therapy. *Best Pract Res Clin Endocrinol Metab*, 17(1):165–175, 2003.

S. R. Davis and J. Tran. Testosterone influences libido and well being in women. *Trends Endocrinol Metab*, 12(1):33–37, 2001.

L.R. Derogatis. *SCL-90-R, administration, scoring & procedures manual-I for the R(evised) version*. Johns Hopkins University School of Medicine: Eigendruck., 1977.

R. Dias, T. W. Robbins, and A. C. Roberts. Dissociation in prefrontal cortex of affective and attentional shifts. *Nature*, 380(6569):69–72, 1996.

Y. C. Ding, H. C. Chi, D. L. Grady, A. Morishima, J. R. Kidd, K. K. Kidd, P. Flodman, M. A. Spence, S. Schuck, J. M. Swanson, Y. P. Zhang, and R. K. Moyzis. Evidence of positive selection acting at the human dopamine receptor d4 gene locus. *Proc Natl Acad Sci U S A*, 99(1):309–314, 2002.

K. Doya. Modulators of decision making. *Nat Neurosci*, 11(4):410–416, 2008.

R. Dunbar. Neocortex size as a constraint on group-size in primates. *J Hum Evol*, 22:469–493, 1992.

R. Dunbar. The social brain hypothesis. *Evol Anthropol*, 6:178–190, 1998.

S. Durston, J. A. Fossella, B. J. Casey, H. E. H. Pol, A. Galvan, H. G. Schnack, M. P. Steenhuis, R. B. Minderaa, J. K. Buitelaar, R. S. Kahn, and H. van Engeland. Differential effects of drd4 and dat1 genotype on fronto-striatal gray matter volumes in a sample of subjects with attention deficit hyperactivity disorder, their unaffected siblings, and controls. *Mol Psychiatry*, 10(7):678–685, 2005.

R. P. Ebstein, O. Novick, R. Umansky, B. Priel, Y. Osher, D. Blaine, E. R. Bennett, L. Nemanov, M. Katz, and R. H. Belmaker. Dopamine d4 receptor (d4dr) exon iii polymorphism associated with the human personality trait of novelty seeking. *Nat Genet*, 12(1):78–80, 1996.

D. A. Edwards. Early androgen stimulation and aggressive behavior in male and female mice. *Physiol Behav*, 4(3):333–338, 1969.

J. Ehrenkranz, E. Bliss, and M. H. Sheard. Plasma testosterone: correlation with aggressive behavior and social dominance in man. *Psychosom Med*, 36(6):469–475, 1974.

J. D. Elsworth and R. H. Roth. Dopamine synthesis, uptake, metabolism, and receptors: relevance to gene therapy of parkinson's disease. *Exp Neurol*, 144(1): 4–9, 1997.

G. M. Everett and J. W. Borcherding. L-dopa: effect on concentrations of dopamine, norepinephrine, and serotonin in brains of mice. *Science*, 168(933):847–850, 1970.

S. V. Faraone, A. E. Doyle, E. Mick, and J. Biederman. Meta-analysis of the association between the 7-repeat allele of the dopamine d-4 receptor gene and attention deficit hyperactivity disorder. *Am J Psychiatry*, 158(7):1052–1057, 2001.

S. V. Faraone, R. H. Perlis, A. E. Doyle, J. W. Smoller, J. J. Goralnick, M. A. Holmgren, and P. Sklar. Molecular genetics of attention-deficit/hyperactivity disorder. *Biol Psychiatry*, 57(11):1313–1323, 2005.

E. C. Finger, A. Marsh, B. Buzas, N. Kamel, R. Rhodes, M. Vythilingham, D. S. Pine, D. Goldman, and J. R. Blair. The impact of tryptophan depletion and 5-httlpr genotype on passive avoidance and response reversal instrumental learning tasks. *Neuropsychopharmacology*, 32(1):206–215, 2007.

U. Fischbacher. z-tree: zurich toolbox for ready-made economic experiments. *Exper Econ*, 10(2):171–178, 2007.

P. B. Fitzgerald, T. L. Brown, and Z. J. Daskalakis. The application of transcranial magnetic stimulation in psychiatry and neurosciences research. *Acta Psychiatr Scand*, 105(5):324–340, 2002.

D. Floden, M. P. Alexander, C. S. Kubu, D. Katz, and D. T. Stuss. Impulsivity and risk-taking behavior in focal frontal lobe lesions. *Neuropsychologia*, 46(1):213–223, 2008.

E. E. Forbes, S. M. Brown, M. Kimak, R. E. Ferrell, S. B. Manuck, and A. R. Hariri. Genetic variation in components of dopamine neurotransmission impacts ventral striatal reactivity associated with impulsivity. *Mol Psychiatry*, 14(1):60–70, 2009.

J. H. Friedman. Punding on levodopa. *Biol Psychiatry*, 36(5):350–351, 1994.

S. J. Gatley, D. Pan, R. Chen, G. Chaturvedi, and Y. S. Ding. Affinities of methylphenidate derivatives for dopamine, norepinephrine and serotonin transporters. *Life Sci*, 58(12):231–239, 1996.

M. S. George, Z. Nahas, F. A. Kozel, X. Li, S. Denslow, K. Yamanaka, A. Mishory, M. J. Foust, and D. E. Bohning. Mechanisms and state of the art of transcranial magnetic stimulation. *J ECT*, 18(4):170–181, 2002.

W. Gerschlager, H. R. Siebner, and J. C. Rothwell. Decreased corticospinal excitability after subthreshold 1 hz rtms over lateral premotor cortex. *Neurology*, 57(3): 449–55, 2001.

L. R. R. Gianotti, D. Knoch, P. L. Faber, D. Lehmann, R. D. Pascual-Marqui, C. Diezi, C. Schoch, C. Eisenegger, and E. Fehr. Tonic activity level in the right prefrontal cortex predicts individuals' risk taking. *Psychol Sci*, 20(1):33–38, 2009.

A. Gjedde, J. Reith, S. Dyve, G. Lger, M. Guttman, M. Diksic, A. Evans, and H. Kuwabara. Dopa decarboxylase activity of the living human brain. *Proc Natl Acad Sci U S A*, 88(7):2721–2725, 1991.

F. Gonon. The dopaminergic hypothesis of attention-deficit/hyperactivity disorder needs re-examining. *Trends Neurosci*, 32(1):2–8, 2009.

J. A. Gorski, S. A. Balogh, J. M. Wehner, and K. R. Jones. Learning deficits in forebrain-restricted brain-derived neurotrophic factor mutant mice. *Neuroscience*, 121(2):341–354, 2003.

A. M. Gotham, R. G. Brown, and C. D. Marsden. Levodopa treatment may benefit or impair frontal function in parkinsons-disease. *Lancet*, 2(8513):970–971, 1986.

A. M. Gotham, R. G. Brown, and C. D. Marsden. Frontal cognitive function in patients with parkinson's disease 'on' and 'off' levodopa. *Brain*, 111 (Pt 2):299–321, 1988.

D. A. Granger, E. A. Shirtcliff, A. Booth, K. T. Kivlighan, and E. B. Schwartz. The "trouble" with salivary testosterone. *Psychoneuroendocrinology*, 29(10):1229–1240, 2004.

V. J. Grant and J. T. France. Dominance and testosterone in women. *Biol Psychol*, 58(1):41–47, 2001.

P. B. Grino, J. E. Griffin, and J. D. Wilson. Testosterone at high concentrations interacts with the human androgen receptor similarly to dihydrotestosterone. *Endocrinology*, 126(2):1165–1172, 1990.

W. Gueth, R. Schmittberger, and B. Schwarze. An experimental analysis of ultimatum bargaining. *J Econ Behav Organ*, 3:367–388, 1982.

M. Hallett. Transcranial magnetic stimulation and the human brain. *Nature*, 406 (6792):147–150, 2000.

M. Hallett. Transcranial magnetic stimulation: A primer. *Neuron*, 55(2):187–199, 2007.

A. Hamidovic, U. J. Kang, and H. de Wit. Effects of low to moderate acute doses of pramipexole on impulsivity and cognition in healthy volunteers. *J Clin Psychopharmacol*, 28(1):45–51, 2008.

J. A. Harris, P. A. Vernon, and D. I. Boomsma. The heritability of testosterone: A study of dutch adolescent twins and their parents. *Behav Genet*, 28(3):165–171, 1998.

A. Heinz, D. Goldman, D. W. Jones, R. Palmour, D. Hommer, J. G. Gorey, K. S. Lee, M. Linnoila, and D. R. Weinberger. Genotype influences in vivo dopamine transporter availability in human striatum. *Neuropsychopharmacology*, 22(2): 133–9, 2000.

D. H. Hellhammer. *Stress: the brain-body connection*. S. Karger, Basel, 2008.

J. Henrich, R. Boyd, S. Bowles, C. Camerer, E. Fehr, H. Gintis, R. McElreath, M. Alvard, A. Barr, J. Ensminger, N. S. Henrich, K. Hill, F. Gil-White, M. Gurven, F. W. Marlowe, J. Q. Patton, and D. Tracer. Economic man in cross-cultural perspective: Behavioral experiments in 15 small-scale societies. *Behav Brain Sci*, 28(6): 795–855, 2005.

E. J. Hermans, P. Putman, J. M. Baas, H. P. Koppeschaar, and J. van Honk. A single administration of testosterone reduces fear-potentiated startle in humans. *Biol Psychiatry*, 59(9):872–874, 2006a.

E. J. Hermans, P. Putman, and J. van Honk. Testosterone administration reduces empathetic behavior: a facial mimicry study. *Psychoneuroendocrinology*, 31(August):859–866, 2006b.

E. J. Hermans, N. F. Ramsey, and J. van Honk. Exogenous testosterone enhances responsiveness to social threat in the neural circuitry of social aggression in humans. *Biol Psychiatry*, 63(3):263–270, 2008.

R. Hertwig and A. Ortmann. Experimental practices in economics: A methodological challenge for psychologists? *Behav Brain Sci*, 24(3):383–389, 2001.

BIBLIOGRAPHY

C. C. Hilgetag, H. Theoret, and A. Pascual-Leone. Enhanced visual spatial attention ipsilateral to rtms-induced 'virtual lesions' of human parietal cortex. *Nat Neurosci*, 4(9):953–957, 2001.

F. Hirayama and K. Uekama. Cyclodextrin-based controlled drug release system. *Adv Drug Deliv Rev*, 36(1):125–141, 1999.

E. Hoffman, K. McCabe, K. Shachat, and V. Smith. Preferences, property rights, and anonymity in bargaining games. *Games Econ Behav*, 7:346–380, 1994.

U. Hoffrage, A. Weber, R. Hertwig, and V. M. Chase. How to keep children safe in traffic: Find the daredevils early. *J Exp Psychol Appl*, 9(4):249–260, 2003.

F. T. Husain, G. Nandipati, A. R. Braun, L. G. Cohen, M. A. Tagamets, and B. Horwitz. Simulating transcranial magnetic stimulation during pet with a large-scale neural network model of the prefrontal cortex and the visual system. *Neuroimage*, 15(1):58–73, 2002.

Kent E Hutchison, John McGeary, Andrew Smolen, Angela Bryan, and Robert M Swift. The drd4 vntr polymorphism moderates craving after alcohol consumption. *Health Psychol*, 21(2):139–146, 2002.

H. Ito, H. Takahashi, R. Arakawa, H. Takano, and T. Suhara. Normal database of dopaminergic neurotransmission system in human brain measured by positron emission tomography. *Neuroimage*, 39(2):555–565, 2008.

R. Jalinous. Technical and practical aspects of magnetic nerve stimulation. *J Clin Neurophysiol*, 8(1):10–25, 1991.

J. A. Johnson, A. P. Strafella, and R. J. Zatorre. The role of the dorsolateral prefrontal cortex in bimodal divided attention: two transcranial magnetic stimulation studies. *J Cogn Neurosci*, 19(6):907–920, 2007.

R. A. Josephs, M. L. Newman, R. P. Brown, and J. M. Beer. Status, testosterone, and human intellectual performance: stereotype threat as status concern. *Psychol Sci*, 14(2):158–163, 2003.

R. A. Josephs, J. G. Sellers, M. L. Newman, and P. H. Mehta. The mismatch effect: when testosterone and status are at odds. *J Pers Soc Psychol*, 90(6):999–1013, 2006.

M. Jueptner and C. Weiller. Review: does measurement of regional cerebral blood flow reflect synaptic activity? implications for pet and fmri. *Neuroimage*, 2(2): 148–156, 1995.

F. Kagitani, S. Uchida, H. Hotta, and A. Sato. Effects of nicotine on blood flow and delayed neuronal death following intermittent transient ischemia in rat hippocampus. *Jpn J Physiol*, 50(6):585–595, 2000.

F. J. Karsch. Central actions of ovarian steroids in the feedback regulation of pulsatile secretion of luteinizing hormone. *Annu Rev Physiol*, 49:365–382, 1987.

E. B. Keverne, F. L. Martel, and C. M. Nevison. Primate brain evolution: genetic and functional considerations. *Proc Biol Sci*, 263(1371):689–696, 1996.

T. A. Kimbrell, R. T. Dunn, M. S. George, A. L. Danielson, M. W. Willis, J. D. Repella, B. E. Benson, P. Herscovitch, R. M. Post, and E. M. Wassermann. Left prefrontal-repetitive transcranial magnetic stimulation (rtms) and regional cerebral glucose metabolism in normal volunteers. *Psychiatry Res*, 115(3):101–113, 2002.

C. Kirschbaum and D. H. Hellhammer. Salivary cortisol in psychoneuroendocrine research - recent developments and applications. *Psychoneuroendocrinology*, 19 (4):313–333, 1994.

S. J. Kish, K. Shannak, and O. Hornykiewicz. Uneven pattern of dopamine loss in the striatum of patients with idiopathic parkinson's disease. pathophysiologic and clinical implications. *N Engl J Med*, 318(14):876–880, 1988.

A. N. Kluger, Z. Siegfried, and R. P. Ebstein. A meta-analysis of the association between drd4 polymorphism and novelty seeking. *Mol Psychiatry*, 7(7):712–717, 2002.

D. Knoch and E. Fehr. Resisting the power of temptations: the right prefrontal cortex and self-control. *Ann N Y Acad Sci*, 1104:123–134, 2007.

D. Knoch, L. R. Gianotti, A. Pascual-Leone, V. Treyer, M. Regard, M. Hohmann, and P. Brugger. Disruption of right prefrontal cortex by low-frequency repetitive transcranial magnetic stimulation induces risk-taking behavior. *J Neurosci*, 26 (24):6469–6472, 2006a.

D. Knoch, A. Pascual-Leone, K. Meyer, V. Treyer, and E. Fehr. Diminishing reciprocal fairness by disrupting the right prefrontal cortex. *Science*, 314(5800):829–832, 2006b.

BIBLIOGRAPHY

D. Knoch, V. Treyer, M. Regard, R. M. Muri, A. Buck, and B. Weber. Lateralized and frequency-dependent effects of prefrontal rtms on regional cerebral blood flow. *Neuroimage*, 31(2):641–648, 2006c.

A. Kondacs and M. Szab. Long-term intra-individual variability of the background eeg in normals. *Clin Neurophysiol*, 110(10):1708–1716, 1999.

I. J. Kopin. Catecholamine metabolism: basic aspects and clinical significance. *Pharmacol Rev*, 37(4):333–364, 1985.

M. Kosfeld, M. Heinrichs, P. J. Zak, U. Fischbacher, and E. Fehr. Oxytocin increases trust in humans. *Nature*, 435(7042):673–676, 2005.

S. M. Kosslyn, A. Pascual-Leone, O. Felician, S. Camposano, J. P. Keenan, W. L. Thompson, G. Ganis, K. E. Sukel, and N. M. Alpert. The role of area 17 in visual imagery: convergent evidence from pet and rtms. *Science*, 284(5411):167–70, 1999.

L. S. Krimer, E. C. Muly, G. V. Williams, and P. S. Goldman-Rakic. Dopaminergic regulation of cerebral cortical microcirculation. *Nat Neurosci*, 1(4):286–289, 1998.

R. Kuczenski and D. S. Segal. Effects of methylphenidate on extracellular dopamine, serotonin, and norepinephrine: comparison with amphetamine. *J Neurochem*, 68(5):2032–2037, 1997.

R. Ladouceur, D. Dub, and A. Bujold. Prevalence of pathological gambling and related problems among college students in the quebec metropolitan area. *Can J Psychiatry*, 39(5):289–293, 1994.

R. A. Lahti, R. C. Roberts, E. V. Cochrane, R. J. Primus, D. W. Gallager, and C. A. Tamminga. [h-3]-ngd-94-1 binding in human postmortem brain of normals and schizophrenics off-, or on-antipsychotic drugs at death. *Schizophr Res*, 24(1-2): 35–35, 1997.

F. Lanau, M. T. Zenner, O. Civelli, and D. S. Hartman. Epinephrine and norepinephrine act as potent agonists at the recombinant human dopamine d4 receptor. *J Neurochem*, 68(2):804–812, 1997.

A. D. Landman, L. M. Sanford, B. E. Howland, C. Dawes, and E. T. Pritchard. Testosterone in human saliva. *Experientia*, 32(7):940–941, 1976.

K. Langley, L. Marshall, M. van den Bree, H. Thomas, M. Owen, M. O'Donovan, and A. Thapar. Association of the dopamine d4 receptor gene 7-repeat allele with neuropsychological test performance of children with adhd. *Am J Psychiatry*, 161 (1):133–138, 2004.

L. Laux. *State-Trait-Angstinventar : theoretische Grundlagen und Handanweisung.* Beltz Testgesellschaft, Weinheim, [deutsche ausgabe] / edition, 1981.

H. R. Lesieur and S. B. Blume. The south oaks gambling screen (sogs): a new instrument for the identification of pathological gamblers. *Am J Psychiatry*, 144 (9):1184–1188, 1987.

J. Lewald, H. Foltys, and R. Topper. Role of the posterior parietal cortex in spatial hearing. *J Neurosci*, 22(3):RC207, 2002.

D. Li, P. C. Sham, M. J. Owen, and L. He. Meta-analysis shows significant association between dopamine system genes and attention deficit hyperactivity disorder (adhd). *Hum Mol Genet*, 15(14):2276–2284, 2006.

J. B. Lichter, C. L. Barr, J. L. Kennedy, H. H. M. Vantol, K. K. Kidd, and K. J. Livak. A hypervariable segment in the human dopamine receptor d(4) (drd4) gene. *Hum Mol Genet*, 2(6):767–773, 1993.

M. S. Lidow, F. Wang, Y. Cao, and P. S. Goldman-Rakic. Layer v neurons bear the majority of mrnas encoding the five distinct dopamine receptor subtypes in the primate prefrontal cortex. *Synapse*, 28(1):10–20, 1998.

K. G. Lloyd and O. Hornykiewicz. Occurrence and distribution of aromatic l-amino acid (l-dopa) decarboxylase in the human brain. *J Neurochem*, 19(6):1549–1559, 1972.

G. Loewenstein. Experimental economics from their vantagepoint of behavioural economics. *The Economic Journal*, 109:25–34, 1999.

A. R. Lumia, K. M. Thorner, and M. Y. Mcginnis. Effects of chronically high-doses of the anabolic-androgenic steroid, testosterone, on intermale aggression and sexual-behavior in male-rats. *Physiol Behav*, 55(2):331–335, 1994.

J. M. Lusher, C. Chandler, and D. Ball. Dopamine d4 receptor gene (drd4) is associated with novelty seeking (ns) and substance abuse: the saga continues ... *Mol Psychiatry*, 6(5):497–499, 2001.

F. Maeda, J. P. Keenan, J. M. Tormos, H. Topka, and A. Pascual-Leone. Interindividual variability of the modulatory effects of repetitive transcranial magnetic stimulation on cortical excitability. *Exp Brain Res*, 133(4):425–430, 2000.

F. Manes, B. Sahakian, L. Clark, R. Rogers, N. Antoun, M. Aitken, and T. W. Robbins. Decision-making processes following damage to the prefrontal cortex. *Brain*, 125(Pt 3):624–639, 2002.

A. A. Marsh, E. C. Finger, B. Buzas, N. Soliman, R. A. Richell, M. Vythilingham, D. S. Pine, D. Goldman, and R. J. R. Blair. Impaired recognition of fear facial expressions in 5-httlpr s-polymorphism carriers following tryptophan depletion. *Psychopharmacology (Berl)*, 189(3):387–394, 2006.

A. May, H. Kaube, C. Buchel, C. Eichten, M. Rijntjes, M. Juptner, C. Weiller, and H. C. Diener. Experimental cranial pain elicited by capsaicin: a pet study. *Pain*, 74(1):61–66, 1998.

A. Mazur. A biosocial model of status in face-to-face primate groups. *Soc Forces*, 64 (2):377–402, 1985.

A. Mazur. *Biosociology of dominance and deference*. Rowman & Littlefield, Lanham, 2005.

A. Mazur and A. Booth. Testosterone and dominance in men. *Behav Brain Sci*, 21 (3):353–363, 1998.

A. Mazur and T. A. Lamb. Testosterone, status, and mood in human males. *Horm Behav*, 14(3):236–246, 1980.

A. Mazur, A. Booth, and J. M. Dabbs. Testosterone and chess competition. *Soc Psychol Q*, 55(1):70–77, 1992.

K. D. Mccaul, B. A. Gladue, and M. Joppa. Winning, losing, mood, and testosterone. *Horm Behav*, 26(4):486–504, 1992.

B. S. Mcewen. Steroid-hormones - effect on brain-development and function. *Horm Res*, 37:1–10, 1992.

P. H. Mehta and R. A. Josephs. Testosterone change after losing predicts the decision to compete again. *Horm Behav*, 50(5):684–692, 2006.

R. H. Melloni, D. F. Connor, P. T. X. Hang, R. J. Harrison, and C. F. Ferris. Anabolic-androgenic steroid exposure during adolescence and aggressive behavior in golden hamsters. *Physiol Behav*, 61(3):359–364, 1997.

D. B. Miller and J. P. O'Callaghan. Neuroendocrine aspects of the response to stress. *Metabolism*, 51(6 Suppl 1):5–10, 2002.

E. K. Miller and J. D. Cohen. An integrative theory of prefrontal cortex function. *Annu Rev Neurosci*, 24:167–202, 2001.

S. H. Mitchell. Measures of impulsivity in cigarette smokers and non-smokers. *Psychopharmacology (Berl)*, 146(4):455–464, 1999.

J. A. Molina, M. J. Sainz-Artiga, A. Fraile, F. J. Jimenez-Jimenez, C. Villanueva, M. Orti-Pareja, and P. F. Bermejo. Pathologic gambling in parkinson's disease: A behavioral manifestation of pharmacologic treatment? *Mov Disord*, 15(5):869–872, 2000.

R. Y. Moore, A. L. Whone, S. McGowan, and D. J. Brooks. Monoamine neuron innervation of the normal human brain: an 18f-dopa pet study. *Brain Res*, 982(2):137–145, 2003.

K. I. Morley and W. D. Hall. Using pharmacogenetics and pharmacogenomics in the treatment of psychiatric disorders: some ethical and economic considerations. *J Mol Med*, 82(1):21–30, 2004.

F. M. Mottaghy, M. Gangitano, R. Sparing, B. J. Krause, and A. Pascual-Leone. Segregation of areas related to visual working memory in the prefrontal cortex revealed by rtms. *Cereb Cortex*, 12(4):369–375, 2002.

L. Mrzljak, C. Bergson, M. Pappy, R. Huff, R. Levenson, and P. S. GoldmanRakic. Localization of dopamine d4 receptors in gabaergic neurons of the primate brain. *Nature*, 381(6579):245–248, 1996.

W. Muellbacher, U. Ziemann, B. Boroojerdi, and M. Hallett. Effects of low-frequency transcranial magnetic stimulation on motor excitability and basic motor behavior. *Clin Neurophysiol*, 111(6):1002–1007, 2000.

M. N. Muller and R. W. Wrangham. Dominance, aggression and testosterone in wild chimpanzees: a test of the ' challenge hypothesis '. *Anim Behav*, 67:113–123, 2004.

Z. Nahas, M. Lomarev, D. R. Roberts, A. Shastri, J. P. Lorberbaum, C. Teneback, K. McConnell, D. J. Vincent, X. Li, M. S. George, and D. E. Bohning. Unilateral left prefrontal transcranial magnetic stimulation (tms) produces intensity-dependent bilateral effects as measured by interleaved bold fmri. *Biol Psychiatry*, 50(9):712–720, 2001.

M. Naoi, W. Maruyama, T. Takahashi, M. Ota, and H. Parvez. Inhibition of tryptophan hydroxylase by dopamine and the precursor amino acids. *Biochem Pharmacol*, 48(1):207–211, 1994.

M. L. Newman, J. G. Sellers, and R. A. Josephs. Testosterone, cognition, and social status. *Horm Behav*, 47(2):205–211, 2005.

A. Newman-Tancredi, V. Audinot-Bouchez, A. Gobert, and M. J. Millan. Noradrenaline and adrenaline are high affinity agonists at dopamine d4 receptors. *Eur J Pharmacol*, 319(2-3):379–383, 1997.

E. Nieschlag. *Testosterone action, deficiency, substitution*. Cambridge University Press, Cambridge, 3rd ed, reprinted edition, 2006.

H. Norris. Action of sedatives on brain stem oculomotor systems in man. *Neuropharmacology*, 10(2):181–191, 1971.

J. N. Oak, J. Oldenhof, and H. H. M. van Tol. The dopamine d-4 receptor: one decade of research. *Eur J Pharmacol*, 405(1-3):303–327, 2000.

K. N. Ochsner, R. D. Ray, J. C. Cooper, E. R. Robertson, S. Chopra, J. D. Gabrieli, and J. J. Gross. For better or for worse: neural systems supporting the cognitive down- and up-regulation of negative emotion. *Neuroimage*, 23(2):483–499, 2004.

T. Ohnishi, H. Matsuda, E. Imabayashi, S. Okabe, H. Takano, N. Arai, and Y. Ugawa. rcbf changes elicited by rtms over dlpfc in humans. *Suppl Clin Neurophysiol*, 57:715–720, 2004.

J. Oldenhof, R. Vickery, M. Anafi, J. Oak, A. Ray, O. Schoots, T. Pawson, M. von Zastrow, and H. H. Van Tol. Sh3 binding domains in the dopamine d4 receptor. *Biochemistry (Mosc)*, 37(45):15726–15736, 1998.

C. C. Overtoom, M. N. Verbaten, C. Kemner, J. L. Kenemans, H. van Engeland, J. K. Buitelaar, M. W. van der Molen, J. van der Gugten, H. Westenberg, R. A. A. Maes, and H. S. Koelega. Effects of methylphenidate, desipramine, and l-dopa on attention and inhibition in children with attention deficit hyperactivity disorder. *Behav Brain Res*, 145(1-2):7–15, 2003.

W. M. Pardridge and L. J. Mietus. Transport of steroid hormones through the rat blood-brain barrier. primary role of albumin-bound hormone. *J Clin Invest*, 64(1): 145–154, 1979.

A. Pascual-Leone, J. M. Tormos, J. Keenan, F. Tarazona, C. Canete, and M. D. Catala. Study and modulation of human cortical excitability with transcranial magnetic stimulation. *J Clin Neurophysiol*, 15(4):333–343, 1998.

J. H. Patton, M. S. Stanford, and E. S. Barratt. Factor structure of the barratt impulsiveness scale. *J Clin Psychol*, 51(6):768–74, 1995.

I. Perez de Castro, A. Ibanez, P. Torres, J. Saiz-Ruiz, and J. Fernandez-Piqueras. Genetic association study between pathological gambling and a functional dna polymorphism at the d4 receptor gene. *Pharmacogenetics*, 7(5):345–348, 1997.

M. Petrides and D. N. Pandya. Dorsolateral prefrontal cortex: comparative cytoarchitectonic analysis in the human and the macaque brain and corticocortical connection patterns. *Eur J Neurosci*, 11(3):1011–1036, 1999.

D. W. Pfaff. Patterns of steroid hormone effects on electrical and molecular events in hypothalamic neurons. *Mol Neurobiol*, 3(3):135–154, 1989.

M. Pirmohamed. Pharmacogenetics and pharmacogenomics. *Br J Clin Pharmacol*, 52(4):345–347, 2001.

M. Pirmohamed and B. K. Park. Genetic susceptibility to adverse drug reactions. *Trends Pharmacol Sci*, 22(6):298–305, 2001.

R.A. Poldrack. Can cognitive processes be inferred from neuroimaging data? *Trends Cogn Sci*, 10(2):59–63, 2006.

H. G. Pope and D. L. Katz. Affective and psychotic symptoms associated with anabolic steroid use. *Am J Psychiatry*, 145(4):487–490, 1988.

H. G. Pope and D. L. Katz. Homicide and near-homicide by anabolic-steroid users. *J Clin Psychiatry*, 51(1):28–31, 1990.

H. G. Pope, E. M. Kouri, and J. I. Hudson. Effects of supraphysiologic doses of testosterone on mood and aggression in normal men: a randomized controlled trial. *Arch Gen Psychiatry*, 57(2):133–140, 2000.

BIBLIOGRAPHY

O. Prante, R. Tietze, C. Hocke, S. Loeber, H. Huebner, T. Kuwert, and P. Gmeiner. Synthesis, radiofluorination, and in vitro evaluation of pyrazolo[1,5-a]pyridine-based dopamine d4 receptor ligands: discovery of an inverse agonist radioligand for pet. *J Med Chem*, 51(6):1800–1810, 2008.

R. J. Primus, A. Thurkauf, J. Xu, E. Yevich, S. McInerney, K. Shaw, J. F. Tallman, and D. W. Gallager. Localization and characterization of dopamine d-4 binding sites in rat and human brain by use of the novel, d-4 receptor-selective ligand [h-3]ngd 94-1 .2. *J Pharmacol Exp Ther*, 282(2):1020–1027, 1997.

L. Prockop, S. Fahn, and P. Barbour. Homovanillic acid: entry rate kinetics for transfer from plasma to cerebrospinal fluid. *Brain Res*, 80(3):435–442, 1974.

F. E. Purifoy and L. H. Koopmans. Androstenedione, testosterone, and free testosterone concentration in women of various occupations. *Soc Biol*, 26(3):179–188, 1979.

S. Rahman, B. J. Sahakia, R. N. Cardinal, R. Rogers, and T. W. Robbins. Decision making and neuropsychiatry. *Trends Cogn Sci*, 5(6):271–277, 2001.

N. Raylu and T. P. S. Oei. Pathological gambling. a comprehensive review. *Clin Psychol Rev*, 22(7):1009–1061, 2002.

D. Riad-Fahmy, G. F. Read, R. F. Walker, S. M. Walker, and K. Griffiths. Determination of ovarian steroid hormone levels in saliva. an overview. *J Reprod Med*, 32 (4):254–272, 1987.

J. Riba, U. K. Kraemer, M. Heldmann, S. Richter, and T. M. Muente. Dopamine agonist increases risk taking but blunts reward-related brain activity. *PLoS ONE*, 3(6):e2479, 2008.

R. M. Ridley and H. F. Baker. Stereotypy in monkeys and humans. *Psychol Med*, 12(1):61–72, 1982.

A. Rivera, B. Cullar, F. J. Girn, D. K. Grandy, A. de la Calle, and R. Moratalla. Dopamine d4 receptors are heterogeneously distributed in the striosomes/matrix compartments of the striatum. *J Neurochem*, 80(2):219–229, 2002.

E. M. Robertson, J. M. Tormos, F. Maeda, and A. Pascual-Leone. The role of the dorsolateral prefrontal cortex during sequence learning is specific for spatial information. *Cereb Cortex*, 11(7):628–635, 2001.

E. M. Robertson, H. Theoret, and A. Pascual-Leone. Studies in cognition: the problems solved and created by transcranial magnetic stimulation. *J Cogn Neurosci*, 15(7):948–960, 2003.

R. D. Rogers, A. M. Owen, H. C. Middleton, E. J. Williams, J. D. Pickard, B. J. Sahakian, and T. W. Robbins. Choosing between small, likely rewards and large, unlikely rewards activates inferior and orbital prefrontal cortex. *J Neurosci*, 19(20):9029–9038, 1999.

J. P. Roiser, A. D. Blackwell, R. Cools, L. Clark, D. C. Rubinsztein, T. W. Robbins, and B. J. Sahakian. Serotonin transporter polymorphism mediates vulnerability to loss of incentive motivation following acute tryptophan depletion. *Neuropsychopharmacology*, 31(10):2264–2272, 2006.

J. P. Roiser, U. Mueller, L. Clark, and B. S. Sahakian. The effects of acute tryptophan depletion and serotonin transporter polymorphism on emotional processing in memory and attention. *Int J Neuropsychopharmacol*, 10(4):449–461, 2007.

T. Roman, M. Schmitz, G. Polanczyk, M. Eizirik, L. A. Rohde, and M. H. Hutz. Attention-deficit hyperactivity disorder: A study of association with both the dopamine transporter gene and the dopamine d4 receptor gene. *Am J Med Genet*, 105(5):471–478, 2001.

J. R. Romero, D. Anschel, R. Sparing, M. Gangitano, and A. Pascual-Leone. Subthreshold low frequency repetitive transcranial magnetic stimulation selectively decreases facilitation in the motor cortex. *Clin Neurophysiol*, 113(1):101–107, 2002.

R. M. Rose, J. W. Holaday, and I. S. Bernstei. Plasma testosterone, dominance rank and aggressive behaviour in male rhesus monkeys. *Nature*, 231(5302):366–372, 1971.

A. Rotem and E. Moses. Magnetic stimulation of one-dimensional neuronal cultures. *Biophys J*, 94(12):5065–5078, 2008.

R. Rowe, B. Maughan, C. M. Worthman, E. J. Costello, and A. Angold. Testosterone, antisocial behavior, and social dominance in boys: Pubertal development and biosocial interaction. *Biol Psychiatry*, 55(5):546–552, 2004.

M. Rubinstein, T. J. Phillips, J. R. Bunzow, T. L. Falzone, G. Dziewczapolski, G. Zhang, Y. Fang, J. L. Larson, J. A. McDougall, J. A. Chester, C. Saez, T. A.

Pugsley, O. Gershanik, M. J. Low, and D. K. Grandy. Mice lacking dopamine d4 receptors are supersensitive to ethanol, cocaine, and methamphetamine. *Cell*, 90 (6):991–1001, 1997.

J. S. Rubinsztein, P. C. Fletcher, R. D. Rogers, L. W. Ho, F. I. Aigbirhio, E. S. Paykel, T. W. Robbins, and B. J. Sahakian. Decision-making in mania: a pet study. *Brain*, 124(Pt 12):2550–2563, 2001.

G. Rylander. Psychoses and the punding and choreiform syndromes in addiction to central stimulant drugs. *Psychiatr Neurol Neurochir*, 75(3):203–212, 1972.

A. T. Sack and D. E. Linden. Combining transcranial magnetic stimulation and functional imaging in cognitive brain research: possibilities and limitations. *Brain Res Brain Res Rev*, 43(1):41–56, 2003.

A. T. Sack, J. A. Camprodon, A. Pascual-Leone, and R. Goebel. The dynamics of interhemispheric compensatory processes in mental imagery. *Science*, 308(5722): 702–704, 2005.

A. T. Sack, A. Kohler, S. Bestmann, D. E. Linden, P. Dechent, R. Goebel, and J. Baudewig. Imaging the brain activity changes underlying impaired visuospatial judgments: Simultaneous fmri, tms, and behavioral studies. *Cereb Cortex*, 2007.

M. Sakagami and X. Pan. Functional role of the ventrolateral prefrontal cortex in decision making. *Curr Opin Neurobiol*, 17(2):228–233, 2007.

A. G. Sanfey, J. K. Rilling, J. A. Aronson, L. E. Nystrom, and J. D. Cohen. The neural basis of economic decision-making in the ultimatum game. *Science*, 300 (5626):1755–1758, 2003.

R. J. Santen and C. W. Bardin. Episodic luteinizing hormone secretion in man. pulse analysis, clinical interpretation, physiologic mechanisms. *J Clin Invest*, 52 (10):2617–2628, 1973.

R. M. Sapolsky. Testicular function, social rank and personality among wild baboons. *Psychoneuroendocrinology*, 16(4):281–293, 1991.

A. Sato, Y. Sato, and S. Uchida. Regulation of regional cerebral blood flow by cholinergic fibers originating in the basal forebrain. *Int J Dev Neurosci*, 19(3):327–337, 2001.

O. Schoots and H. H. M. Van Tol. The human dopamine d4 receptor repeat sequences modulate expression. *Pharmacogenomics J*, 3(6):343–348, 2003.

D. Schultheiss and C. G. Stief. Highlighting 70 years of testosterone substitution. *Eur Urol*, 4(6):1–3, 2005.

O. C. Schultheiss, K. L. Campbell, and D. C. McClelland. Implicit power motivation moderates men's testosterone responses to imagined and real dominance success. *Horm Behav*, 36(3):234–241, 1999.

W. Schultz, P. Dayan, and P. R. Montague. A neural substrate of prediction and reward. *Science*, 275(5306):1593–1599, 1997.

P. Schwenkmezger, V. Hodapp, and C. D. Spielberger. *Das State-Trait-Aergerausdruck-Inventar STAXI [The State-Trait Anger Expression Inventory (STAXI)]*. Verlag Hans Huber, Bern, 1992.

P. Seeman, H. C. Guan, H. H. Van Tol, and H. B. Niznik. Low density of dopamine d4 receptors in parkinson's, schizophrenia, and control brain striata. *Synapse*, 14(4):247–253, 1993.

J. G. Sellers, M. R. Mehl, and R. A. Josephs. Hormones and personality: Testosterone as a marker of individual differences. *J Res Pers*, 41(1):126–138, 2007.

S. Sen, R. M. Nesse, S. F. Stoltenberg, S. Li, L. Gleiberman, A. Chakravarti, A. B. Weder, and M. Burmeister. A bdnf coding variant is associated with the neo personality inventory domain neuroticism, a risk factor for depression. *Neuropsychopharmacology*, 28(2):397–401, 2003.

H. R. Siebner and J. Rothwell. Transcranial magnetic stimulation: new insights into representational cortical plasticity. *Exp Brain Res*, 148(1):1–16, 2003.

T. Simoncini and A. R. Genazzani. Non-genomic actions of sex steroid hormones. *Eur J Endocrinol*, 148(3):281–292, 2003.

P. Slovic. Risk-taking in children - age and sex differences. *Child Dev*, 37(1):169–175, 1966.

M. H. Sohn, S. Ursu, J. R. Anderson, V. A. Stenger, and C. S. Carter. Inaugural article: the role of prefrontal cortex and posterior parietal cortex in task switching. *Proc Natl Acad Sci U S A*, 97(24):13448–13453, 2000.

S. M. Specker, G. A. Carlson, G. A. Christenson, and M. Marcotte. Impulse control disorders and attention deficit disorder in pathological gamblers. *Ann Clin Psychiatry*, 7(4):175–179, 1995.

A. M. Speer, M. W. Willis, P. Herscovitch, M. Daube-Witherspoon, J. R. Shelton, B. E. Benson, R. M. Post, and E. M. Wassermann. Intensity-dependent regional cerebral blood flow during 1-hz repetitive transcranial magnetic stimulation (rtms) in healthy volunteers studied with h2150 positron emission tomography: I. effects of primary motor cortex rtms. *Biol Psychiatry*, 54(8):818–825, 2003.

Z. Steel and A. Blaszczynski. Impulsivity, personality disorders and pathological gambling severity. *Addiction*, 93(6):895–905, 1998.

R. Steyer, P. Schwenkmezger, P. Notz, and M. Eid. *Der Mehrdimensionale Befindlichkeitsfragebogen (MDBF) [Multidimensional Mood State Questionnaire]*. Hogrefe, Gttingen, 1997.

C. A. Stuenkel, R. E. Dudley, and S. S. Yen. Sublingual administration of testosterone-hydroxypropyl-beta-cyclodextrin inclusion complex simulates episodic androgen release in hypogonadal men. *J Clin Endocrinol Metab*, 72 (5):1054–1009, 1991.

A. L. Svingos, S. Periasamy, and V. M. Pickel. Presynaptic dopamine d(4) receptor localization in the rat nucleus accumbens shell. *Synapse*, 36(3):222–232, 2000.

R. Swainson, R. D. Rogers, B. J. Sahakian, B. A. Summers, C. E. Polkey, and T. W. Robbins. Probabilistic learning and reversal deficits in patients with parkinson's disease or frontal or temporal lobe lesions: possible adverse effects of dopaminergic medication. *Neuropsychologia*, 38(5):596–612, 2000.

J. M. Swanson, M. Kinsbourne, J. Nigg, B. Lanphear, G. A. Stefanatos, N. Volkow, E. Taylor, B. J. Casey, F. X. Castellanos, and P. D. Wadhwa. Etiologic subtypes of attention-deficit/hyperactivity disorder: brain imaging, molecular genetic and environmental factors and the dopamine hypothesis. *Neuropsychol Rev*, 17(1): 39–59, 2007.

J. P. Tangney, R. F. Baumeister, and A. L. Boone. High self-control predicts good adjustment, less pathology, better grades, and interpersonal success. *J Pers*, 72 (2):271–324, 2004.

G. W. Thickbroom. Transcranial magnetic stimulation and synaptic plasticity: experimental framework and human models. *Exp Brain Res*, 180(4):583–93, 2007.

A. J. Tilbrook, A. I. Turner, and I. J. Clarke. Effects of stress on reproduction in nonrodent mammals: the role of glucocorticoids and sex differences. *Rev Reprod*, 5(2):105–113, 2000.

A. Tuiten, J. Van Honk, H. Koppeschaar, C. Bernaards, J. Thijssen, and R. Verbaten. Time course of effects of testosterone administration on sexual arousal in women. *Arch Gen Psychiatry*, 57(2):149–153, 2000.

A. Tuiten, J. van Honk, R. Verbaten, E. Laan, W. Everaerd, and H. Stam. Can sublingual testosterone increase subjective and physiological measures of laboratory-induced sexual arousal? *Arch Gen Psychiatry*, 59(5):465–466, 2002.

S. Uchida, F. Kagitani, H. Nakayama, and A. Sato. Effect of stimulation of nicotinic cholinergic receptors on cortical cerebral blood flow and changes in the effect during aging in anesthetized rats. *Neurosci Lett*, 228(3):203–206, 1997.

J. R. Udry and L. M. Talbert. Sex-hormone effects on personality at puberty. *J Pers Soc Psychol*, 54(2):291–295, 1988.

J. R. Udry, N. M. Morris, and J. Kovenock. Androgen effects on women's gendered behaviour. *J Biosoc Sci*, 27(3):359–368, 1995.

K. van Craenenbroeck, S. D. Clark, M. J. Cox, J. N. Oak, F. Liu, and H. H. M. Van Tol. Folding efficiency is rate-limiting in dopamine d4 receptor biogenesis. *J Biol Chem*, 280(19):19350–19357, 2005.

J. van Honk and D. J. Schutter. Testosterone reduces conscious detection of signals serving social correction: implications for antisocial behavior. *Psychol Sci*, 18(8):663–667, 2007.

J. van Honk, A. Tuiten, R. Verbaten, M. van den Hout, H. Koppeschaar, J. Thijssen, and E. de Haan. Correlations among salivary testosterone, mood, and selective attention to threat in humans. *Horm Behav*, 36(1):17–24, 1999.

J. van Honk, A. Tuiten, E. Hermans, P. Putman, H. Koppeschaar, J. Thijssen, R. Verbaten, and L. van Doornen. A single administration of testosterone induces cardiac accelerative responses to angry faces in healthy young women. *Behav Neurosci*, 115(1):238–242, 2001.

J. van Honk, D. J. Schutter, E. J. Hermans, P. Putman, A. Tuiten, and H. Koppeschaar. Testosterone shifts the balance between sensitivity for punishment and reward in healthy young women. *Psychoneuroendocrinology*, 29(7): 937–943, 2004.

J. van Honk, J. S. Peper, and D. J. Schutter. Testosterone reduces unconscious fear but not consciously experienced anxiety: implications for the disorders of fear and anxiety. *Biol Psychiatry*, 58(3):218–225, 2005.

H. H. M. van Tol, C. M. Wu, H. C. Guan, K. Ohara, J. R. Bunzow, O. Civelli, J. Kennedy, P. Seeman, H. B. Niznik, and V. Jovanovic. Multiple dopamine-d4 receptor variants in the human-population. *Nature*, 358(6382):149–152, 1992.

A. Verdejo-Garcia, A. J. Lawrence, and L. Clark. Impulsivity as a vulnerability marker for substance-use disorders: Review of findings from high-risk research, problem gamblers and genetic association studies. *Neurosci Biobehav Rev*, 32(4): 777–810, 2008.

V. Viau. Functional cross-talk between the hypothalamic-pituitary-gonadal and - adrenal axes. *J Neuroendocrinol*, 14(6):506–513, 2002.

S. Vijayraghavan, M. Wang, S. G. Birnbaum, G. V. Williams, and A. F. T. Arnsten. Inverted-u dopamine d1 receptor actions on prefrontal neurons engaged in working memory. *Nat Neurosci*, 10(3):376–384, 2007.

D. Voet, J. G. Voet, A. Maelicke, and W. Mueller-Esterl. *Biochemie*. VCH Verlagsgesellschaft, Weinheim, 1992.

V. Voon, M. N. Potenza, and T. Thomsen. Medication-related impulse control and repetitive behaviors in parkinson's disease. *Curr Opin Neurol*, 20(4):484–492, 2007a.

V. Voon, T. Thomsen, J. M. Miyasaki, M. de Souza, A. Shafro, S. H. Fox, S. Duff-Canning, A. E. Lang, and M. Zurowski. Factors associated with dopaminergic drug-related pathological gambling in parkinson disease. *Arch Neurol*, 64(2):212–216, 2007b.

V. Walsh and A. Cowey. Transcranial magnetic stimulation and cognitive neuroscience. *Nat Rev Neurosci*, 1(1):73–79, 2000.

V. Walsh and M. Rushworth. A primer of magnetic stimulation as a tool for neuropsychology. *Neuropsychologia*, 37(2):125–135, 1999.

C. Wang, D. H. Catlin, L. M. Demers, B. Starcevic, and R. S. Swerdloff. Measurement of total serum testosterone in adult men: Comparison of current laboratory methods versus liquid chromatography-tandem mass spectrometry. *J Clin Endocrinol Metab*, 89(2):534–543, 2004.

X. Wang, P. Zhong, and Z. Yan. Dopamine d-4 receptors modulate gabaergic signaling in pyramidal neurons of prefrontal cortex. *J Neurosci*, 22(21):9185–9193, 2002.

E. M. Wassermann, F. R. Wedegaertner, U. Ziemann, M. S. George, and R. Chen. Crossed reduction of human motor cortex excitability by 1-hz transcranial magnetic stimulation. *Neurosci Lett*, 250(3):141–144, 1998.

C. Wedemeyer, J. D. Goutman, M. E. Avale, L. F. Franchini, M. Rubinstein, and D. J. Calvo. Functional activation by central monoamines of human dopamine d-4 receptor polymorphic variants coupled to girk channels in xenopus oocytes. *Eur J Pharmacol*, 562(3):165–173, 2007.

G. Weinbauer, J. Gromoll, M. Simoni, and E. Nieschlag. *Physiologie der Hodenfunktion.* Andrologie. Thieme Verlag, 2000.

P. Werner, N. Hussy, G. Buell, K. A. Jones, and R. A. North. D2, d3, and d4 dopamine receptors couple to g protein-regulated potassium channels in xenopus oocytes. *Mol Pharmacol*, 49(4):656–661, 1996.

G. V. Williams and P. S. Goldmanrakic. Modulation of memory fields by dopamine d1 receptors in prefrontal cortex. *Nature*, 376(6541):572–575, 1995.

A. H. Wong, C. E. Buckle, and H. H. Van Tol. Polymorphisms in dopamine receptors: what do they tell us? *Eur J Pharmacol*, 410(2-3):183–203, 2000.

M. J. Zigmond, F. E. Bloom, S. C. Landis, J. L. Roberts, and L. R. Squire. *Fundamental neuroscience*. Academic Press, San Diego, California, 1999.

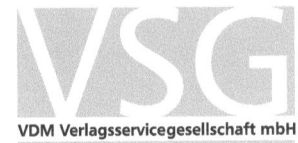

Die VDM Verlagsservicegesellschaft sucht für wissenschaftliche Verlage abgeschlossene und herausragende

Dissertationen, Habilitationen, Diplomarbeiten, Master Theses, Magisterarbeiten usw.

für die kostenlose Publikation als Fachbuch.

Sie verfügen über eine Arbeit, die hohen inhaltlichen und formalen Ansprüchen genügt, und haben Interesse an einer honorarvergüteten Publikation?

Dann senden Sie bitte erste Informationen über sich und Ihre Arbeit per Email an *info@vdm-vsg.de*.

Sie erhalten kurzfristig unser Feedback!

VDM Verlagsservicegesellschaft mbH
Dudweiler Landstr. 99   Telefon +49 681 3720 174
D - 66123 Saarbrücken   Fax   +49 681 3720 1749
www.vdm-vsg.de

Die VDM Verlagsservicegesellschaft mbH vertritt

 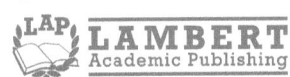 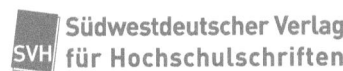

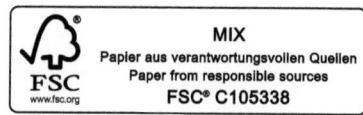

Printed by Books on Demand GmbH, Norderstedt / Germany